Disabled Children Living Away from Home

Dedication

This book is dedicated to two disabled girls whom I cared for many years ago and who left their family homes for foster care in mid-childhood with great emotional distress.

Disabled Children Living Away from Home

in Foster Care and Residential Settings

Edited by Claire Burns

2009
Mac Keith Press
Distributed by Wiley-Blackwell

© 2009 Mac Keith Press

Editor: Hilary M. Hart
Managing Director, Mac Keith Press: Caroline Black
Project Manager: Annalisa Welch
Indexer: Laurence Errington

First published in this edition 2009 by
Mac Keith Press, 6 Market Road, London N7 9PW, UK
British Library Cataloguing-in-Publication data

A catalogue record of this book is available from the British Library

ISBN: 978–1–898683–58–2

Typeset by Keystroke, 28 High Street, Tettenhall, Wolverhampton
Printed by The Lavenham Press Ltd, Water Street, Lavenham, Suffolk
Mac Keith Press is supported by Scope

Contents

Contents

Contributors

Catherine Baines, Retired Civil Servant, Department of Health, UK

Allen Baynes, Education Consultant, Director of Bridge4learning, Shrewbury, UK

Tom Berney, Honorary Consultant Developmental Psychiatrist, Northumberland Tyne & Wear NHS Trust, Newcastle upon Tyne, UK

Claire Burns, Consultant Paediatrician, Community Paediatric Department, Children's Hospital, Oxford, UK

Pat Cawson, Research Consultant on Children's Services and Former Head of Child Protection Research, NSPCC, UK

Jennifer Cousins, *Opening Doors* Disability Project Consultant, British Association for Adoption & Fostering (BAAF), Birmingham, UK

Annette Hames, Consultant Clinical Psychologist, Newcastle Community Team Learning Disability, Northumberland Tyne and Wear NHS Trust, Newcastle upon Tyne, UK

Maraline Jones, Clinical Nurse Specialist for Looked After Children, Community Team, Caerphilly, Mid Glamorgan, UK

Thomas Kus, Consultant Paediatrician, Gloucester Royal Hospital, Gloucester, UK

Mary Mather, Medical Director, FACT Project, Parents for Children, London, UK

Contributors

Heather Payne, Senior Lecturer, Department of Child Health and Associate Dean for Educational Support and Disability, School of Postgraduate Medical and Dental Educational, Cardiff University, Cardiff, UK

Mike Searle, Education Psychologist, foster carer and Director of Bridge4learning, Shrewbury, UK

Moira Szilagyi, Associate Professor of Pediatrics, University of Rochester, New York and Medical Director, Starlight Pediatrics, Monroe County Department of Public Health, Rochester, New York, USA

Introduction

Claire Burns

In 2003 the Mac Keith Meetings Committee ran a 2-day workshop on *Disabled Children Living Away from Home* to consider how care for these children might be improved. The following year the Committee organized a conference for health and social care professionals on the same subject at the Royal Society of Medicine. It was following this that the possibility of publishing a book to document the accumulated knowledge and evidence of those who had contributed to the meetings was raised. We hope the book will provide insights into the difficulties these children face and prompt consideration as to how the standard of care we provide for them can be improved.

We decided at the outset not to consider different groups of disabled children separately but rather use the term 'disabled' to include children and young people with a range of physical, cognitive, emotional and social difficulties. Chapter 1 (Jennifer Cousins) clarifies the terms used in the book and considers the different places disabled children may live when they leave the care of their parents.

The vast majority of disabled children in the United Kingdom (UK) live at home with their families and are well looked after. The main reason for leaving the family home is that the parents feel they can no longer care for the child. The need for services to prevent the breakdown of home care, the different care challenges for parents and the changing patterns of disability are dealt with in Chapter 2 (Mary Mather). For some disabled children, it is concerns about neglectful care and abuse which prompt the move from home. However, whatever the reason, leaving home is a cause of emotional distress to the child. A stable and nuturing home life provides the foundation for future mental health and the disabled child leaving home is at increased risk for subsequent mental health problems.

The new placement is more likely to be successful and mental health and behaviour problems avoided, if the child's carers are well matched to the child and have advice and support readily available to them from social care workers, health professionals (specialist community nurses, paediatricians, child and adolescent mental health workers, therapists and the primary care team) and teachers. A number of Chapters (Chapter 3 by Heather Payne, Chapter 4 by Maraline Jones and Chapter 7 by Thomas Kus and and Heather Payne) consider aspects of health service coordination, others (Chapters 5 by Annette Hames and Chapter 6 by Tom Berney) look at behaviour problems and emotional issues and explore ways of promoting good mental health. Chapter 8 (Mike Searle and Allen Baynes) deals with educational matters and highlights the importance of leisure and fun.

Finding out what the disabled child or young person wants (including those with impaired communication) and ensuring, wherever possible, that these needs are addressed, is key to improving the quality of their lives. Practical ways to improve communication with disabled children are covered in Chapter 9 (Catherine Baines). Professionals who establish friendships with disabled children are more likely to be trusted and this in turn may enable the disabled child to feel safe about discussing their feelings and needs and, at times, disclosing abusive experiences. Research has shown that disabled children are more vulnerable to abuse than others, both in their families and away from home; ways of protecting against this are covered in Chapter 10 (Pat Cawson).

Mindful of the need to learn from other countries we have included a chapter on the experience of a paediatrician working with disabled children who live 'out-of-home' in the United States (Chapter 11 by Moira Szilagyi). Although there are many similarities in the way the UK and USA care for disabled children there are some interesting differences too.

In the UK there is little research evidence for planning effective health interventions for disabled children living away from home. We hope that the experience and reflections collected in this book will enable those involved with these children to provide the support and care necessary for them to achieve their potential and to develop into healthy and resilient individuals. We also hope the book will stimulate further research into the needs of this uniquely vulnerable population of children and young people.

Chapter 1

Disabled Children: Pathways to care

Jennifer Cousins

Introduction

This chapter examines some aspects of the lives of disabled children in the community, and the route they take into and through the 'care system'. It begins by clarifying the terms used, and by distinguishing between the social and medical models of disability. It aims particularly to highlight the role of professionals right across the health and social care sector in ensuring that disabled children's right to family life is upheld.

The titles of publications about disabled children immediately demonstrate how marginalized these children can become:

- *Gone Missing?*
- *Still Missing?*
- *Don't Leave Us Out*
- *Seen but not Heard*
- *The Silent Minority*
- *On the Edge*
- *Valued or Forgotten?*

Their invisibility is made worse by the sheer poverty of the research. It is still unfortunately the case that 'information about the numbers of disabled children and their needs is patchy and rather limited' (Stuart and Baines 2004a:18). The whole field is dogged by a lack of data, statistics that do not compare like with like and badly out dated information. There is a particular problem with definitions: under the term 'disability', some research includes children who have solely emotional and behavioural disorders, whereas other research excludes these children; and some studies include children with educational 'special needs' while others do not. There are no recent comprehensive studies. Readers should therefore approach any data given here with caution.

The position of disabled children in relation to the care system is explored under the following headings:

- Children in Need (children in the community);
- children in residential settings;
- children in residential schools;
- children in hospitals and non-social services respite (short-breaks) provision;
- Looked After children: temporary foster care, family-based short-break care and residential care;
- children who need 'permanence'.

Terms

It will become apparent that the distinctions between being Looked After and not Looked After can be crucial. It may be helpful therefore to clarify the legal terms used in this chapter when reference is made to the care system.

- Children in Need are children living in the community with their own families who are defined as being in need of services under Section 17 of the Children Act 1989 (England & Wales). Disabled children come into this category.
- Looked After children refers to all children who are being Looked After away from home by the local authority. Many Looked After children are placed with social services foster carers or in local authority residential care. However, the care of Looked After children can be delegated to other providers of services, with safeguards, such as voluntary organizations and independent fostering or residential providers.
- Some children live away from home in education or health provision, such as boarding schools and hospitals. These children are not Looked After by the local authority, and different (arguably fewer) safeguards apply. They are, however, covered by Children in Need provisions.
- Looked After is the generic term which covers both:
  - voluntary arrangements made with birth parents (under Section 20 Children Act 1989). The local authority does not gain parental responsibility in these circumstances;
  - statutory arrangements such as an interim or full care order (under Sections 31 & 38 Children Act 1989) acquired through a court where the child is deemed to be suffering from (or likely to suffer) significant harm. Either order provides the local authority with parental responsibility but does not remove parents' responsibility.

  A crucial feature of the Looked After system is the regular *statutory reviews* under the Review of Children's Cases Regulations 1991 that ensure that planning is kept focused and child-centred. After the child has been Looked After for 4 months, the question must be raised about planning for permanence – either a permanent return home or through seeking a permanent new family via adoption or fostering.

This measure was introduced in order to combat children drifting in the care system with no real sense of belonging to a family.

- The term 'in care' is often used as shorthand for all children being Looked After by the local authority. Readers will find the term 'in care' used loosely in this chapter unless its legal application is specifically highlighted.

- 'Special needs' has become a catch-all phrase that is largely meaningless in social care. Every person has needs that are special. It is more accurate, and more respectful, to talk of a particular person's 'specific requirements' and to identify what they are. 'Special needs', however, has evolved from 'Special educational needs' which has a clear definition and system of assessment in the Education Act 1996 and its related Code of Practice. The assessment may lead to a 'Statement of Special Educational Need' that identifies the most appropriate educational support. Children are then deemed to be 'statemented' – a label that can serve not only to secure resources, but also to stigmatize. The fact that legislation does not distinguish between disability and special educational needs tends to make definitions of disability even more complex. 'Not all disabled children have special educational needs. Neither. . . are all statemented children disabled.' (Middleton 1992:75). In 1999, schools in England identified 20% of their pupils as having 'some form of special educational needs'. At that time 3% of pupils had actual 'statements' (Department of Health (DH) 2000:73).

Defining disability

The perspective here is that the terms 'impairment' and 'disability' are separate concepts. 'Impairment' is a functional limitation caused by a physical, mental or sensory condition – a definition that highlights the *permanence* of the condition. 'Disability' on the other hand is the inability to take part equally in the normal life of the community *due to physical and social barriers* (Cousins 2006:11).

According to this model, promoted by campaigners like Oliver (1990) and Morris (1995, 1998) people who have impairments are not so much 'disabled' by their impairment as by the way society creates barriers to full participation and opportunity. 'Disability' is therefore a socially defined term rather than a condition inherent in the individual.

The term 'disabled children' is used throughout this chapter with the specific intention of signalling that children who have impairments are 'disabled' by the world around them: by prejudice, marginalization and stigma, as well as inaccessible buildings, transport and leisure facilities.

The Department of Health summarized these definitional problems as follows:

> *Medical classifications of disability are insensitive as a basis for planning services for families. Labels like autism and cerebral palsy cover a wide range of impairments. In fact children with cerebral palsy are likely to be found at every level of severity.*

> *These labels mean that the primary presenting condition is the focus for other services, yet it may not be this condition that is causing the most stress to the family or child. . .Definitions which do not recognize the multiple nature of the disability, the social circumstances of the family and the changing nature of the need for support, will not offer a sufficiently flexible mechanism on which to plan services.*
>
> *(DH 1998:19)*

Disabled children are often regarded as separate from other children. Their impairment becomes their defining feature, and attracts the focus of specialized medical, educational and social work attention: in effect, they *become* their impairment. One of the challenges in thinking about disabled children is to balance the two contradictory themes – that they are 'just children' but with extra requirements. If society values disabled children as having the same basic needs and rights as all children, it must be concerned to ensure that their right to loving and supportive family life is upheld. This chapter shows that this is by no means guaranteed.

Children in Need

Disabled children in the community are, by definition under the Children Act 1989 (England and Wales), Children in Need. Although it is now taken for granted, the specific inclusion of disabled children in the legislation was a significant step forward. Under the Act, local authorities are required to provide a register of all disabled children living within their boundary; an assessment of need; services which minimize the effects of the disability, and opportunities to live 'normal' lives where possible. Disabled children are included fully within the regulatory framework for *all* children, and the following overarching principles apply:

- the child's welfare is paramount;
- the local authority must work in partnership with parents;
- children should be brought up within their own family where at all possible;
- children's wishes and feelings must be ascertained and taken account of;
- the local authority has a corporate responsibility for children (so-called 'corporate parenting'). As the term suggests, this responsibility does not rest solely with the social services department.

These principles are of particular importance for disabled children.

About 3% of all children in the UK are disabled. Most live at home and many have multiple impairments: the average number of impairments experienced by children aged 5 to 15 living at home was 2.6 (DH 1998). Seventeen thousand families in the community are caring for more than one disabled child, and there are 10 000 severely disabled children with a disabled sibling. Poverty is a significant feature of the lives of these families: there are twice the number of disabled children in 'social class 5' households as in 'social class 1'. Entitlement to provision that would be readily available to others (education, housing, play and leisure opportunities) is often subject to assessment (DH 2000:75) and surveys show that these families are often marginalized by agencies and services. For example only 4% of families with a severely disabled child has access to short-break care, as compared with 19% of foster carers who look after such children (Gordon et al 2000:157).

There are more boys with disabilities than girls, especially in the category of severe disability (Office for National Statistics (ONS) 2004), and an increased incidence of impairments among Asian children (Stuart and Baines 2004a). In all settings, disabled children are more likely to be abused than non-disabled children.

Life is not easy for many families of disabled children in the community. The range of difficulties they encounter may contribute to the fact that disabled children are many times more likely to become Looked After than non-disabled children. The Department of Health data show that whereas 5.7% of disabled children in the general population are in care, only 0.6% of the child population as a whole are in care (DH 1998).

Children in residential settings

Many disabled children spend varying amounts of time in residential provision. It will become apparent that there are important differences in the formal arrangements under which children are placed residentially, but here readers are simply reminded of the issues for disabled children cared for away from home whatever their legal status. In essence, all residential care holds risks for disabled children.

Abuse

The seminal report *People Like Us* (Utting 1997) concluded that disabled children in residential establishments are vulnerable to abuse of all kinds, including peer abuse. Miller (2002) claims that disabled children are more than three times as likely to be abused as non-disabled children. The reasons are well known:

- abusers are known to target communities of vulnerable children;
- disabled children have many different carers – the abuser is less easy to pinpoint;
- intimate care is private, and boundaries between appropriate and abusive touching can be deliberately blurred by an abuser;
- children with communication impairments may be unable to disclose abuse;
- the child's main carer and 'interpreter' may be their abuser;
- a disabled child is less likely to be believed;
- the child may be unable to defend her/himself;
- signs of abuse can be mistaken for self-harm or the result of the physical condition/impairment;
- disabled children may have low self-esteem and 'expect no better';
- the disabled child is used to being 'invaded' by legitimate medical procedures and can no longer distinguish between appropriate and inappropriate touching:

> *The medical experiences I had made me very vulnerable to being abused, it just seemed the same as everything else that had been done to me, so I wasn't able to discriminate.*
>
> **(Westcott 1998:130)**

There are strong societal pressures to believe that disabled children cannot possibly be abused or neglected. This is reinforced by the fact that the criminal justice system still fails to prosecute those who abuse disabled children (Stuart and Baines 2004a). This reluctance to accept reality becomes the first breach in the ring of protection that should encircle the child. So a good starting point for all professionals who come into contact with any disabled child in any residential setting is to be able to *think the unthinkable*.

Loss of family life
The second most crucial concern for disabled children living away from home is the risk that they may lose any sense of family life. Disabled children are multiply at risk. Research by the Department of Health shows that children in residential care can become extremely isolated: overall, two-fifths were not visited by their parents and 25% had had no (and some almost no) visits either from or to home. This amounts to a third of children who are very isolated and potentially more vulnerable as a result (DH 1998).

Because of cost and time constraints, the distance between home and residential provision may militate against frequent visits. It is known that the more severe the impairment the further away the specialist provision is likely to be. A child's communication impairment may reduce the chance of other forms of contact being meaningful (telephone calls, letters, e-mail and texting may be unrealistic); and for some learning disabled children who are unable to hold in mind the concept of an absent family, actual face-to-face meetings may be the *only* way they can feel connected.

Typically, visits either of family to school or child to home reduce over time and relationships can seriously weaken. The result can be a dangerous attenuation of connectedness with the family, with all the risks which that holds for identity, self-esteem, 'belonging', future relationships and care in adulthood.

> *Children with disabilities have fewer informal opportunities to make friends and new contacts, and so the family is crucial in helping them to determine their place in the world and for acting as an advocate when required.*
>
> **(Russell 1995:104)**

It goes without saying that where 52-week provision is offered, these risks increase significantly. Multiply disadvantaged children, however well cared for by the establishment, can be cut adrift from their original community. The Human Rights legislation which guarantees children the 'right to family life'; and the Children Act 1989 which promised all disabled children that their welfare is 'paramount' seem likely after all to be failing some children. The mantra 'working in partnership with parents' is more often interpreted as putting the parents' requirements foremost.

Other needs

Contrary to expectation, the general health care of children in residential establishments is not universally good. Although GP intervention was reasonably regular, two-thirds of children surveyed had not seen a dentist in the last year. Few children had been seen by a psychiatrist, psychologist or psychotherapist, 'somewhat disturbing findings given the considerable degree of behaviour difficulties that existed among disabled children in residential care' (DH 1998:16).

> *Alongside the residential care staff a great deal of responsibility was falling upon social workers and GPs for attending to the children's specific needs, but also for safeguarding their general well-being as independent points of contact.*
>
> *(DH 1998:16)*

These are salutary lessons for health and social care personnel. A study in 1996 of the Independent Visitor scheme (set up through the Children Act 1989) showed that, although warmly welcomed by participants, this scheme was scarcely used by local authorities: only 235 young people (of whom a mere 32 were disabled) had an Independent Visitor (Joseph Rowntree Foundation (JRF) 1998). It is to be hoped that the use of this system has expanded.

Children in residential schools

Legal position

Although the available data about numbers is unreliable, there is a significant group of disabled children who live for varying parts of the year in residential establishments funded by education. The crucial issue here is that although afforded the general protection of any child, and subject to entitlements as Children in Need because of their disability, these children are not regarded as Looked After by the local authority. This is an anomaly fiercely challenged by all the staunchest advocates for disabled children – see in particular Morris (1995, 1998), and Morris et al (2002).

As children in boarding schools are not protected as Looked After children under the Review Regulations 1991, there is a risk that their overall well-being will not be monitored. All establishments have a duty under Section 85 of the Children Act 1989 to notify social services (the 'responsible authority') if a child is living with them for more than 3 months. The responsible authority then has a duty to:

> *. . . take all reasonably practicable steps to enable them to decide whether the child's welfare is adequately safeguarded and promoted while he stays in the accommodation and to decide whether it is necessary to exercise any of their functions under the Act.*
>
> *(DH 1991b:39)*

But, despite 'corporate parenting', the follow-up scrutiny by the 'responsible authority' is widely acknowledged to be patchy and less than rigorous. There is therefore considerable concern that children whose general well-being is not regularly examined by an Independent Reviewing Officer may become cut-off from home and lose their right to family life.

Parental choice
One of the reasons why some children are specifically placed in education rather than social services residential provision by their parents is precisely to avoid the common stigma attached to being in care. Many parents do not wish to be seen to transfer the day to day care of their child to 'the authorities'. While a boarding school is socially acceptable, having your child in care is not. Guilt, fear and a wish to retain control are at the root of this.

The possibility therefore exists that where the parents' and the child's needs do not coincide, the parents' view will naturally prevail. In some extreme instances, the parents' need for respite can take precedence over the child's need for family life. Some commentators argue that extensive use of boarding provision is social care masquerading as education. All the risks outlined above for all residential establishments can obtain.

Risks to children
It has been highlighted that all children living for extended periods away from home are at risk of losing their families. This is supported by research as far back as the seminal *Patterns and Outcomes* collection (DH 1991a), and by the more recent work of Russell (1995). Of even greater concern is that no new permanent family may ever be sought for these children unless challenges are made to the status quo.

Where disabled children fall outside the Looked After provisions, there is no Independent Reviewing Officer asking the required question about 'permanence'. But even where the child is Looked After, this question may not be raised. It is rarely in the mindset of professionals who work with Children in Need and their families to wonder if residential provision might ultimately constitute 'significant harm' even though care by rota and chronic loss of family contact is known to be damaging for children. Staff in children's disabilities teams, feeling deskilled at child protection, may tend to see their job primarily as supporting parents, not challenging them with painful choices about alternative families. And at the back of everyone's mind is the fear that new families may not come forward for disabled children.

Children in hospitals and non-social services respite (short-break) provision
Long-stay hospitals can be used to offer short breaks as respite for families. These are normally NHS provision and fall outside social services scrutiny; they are also more acceptable to parents. The data for this group of vulnerable children are lacking:

> *Current available data on admissions into health care settings does not identify disabled children as a group for whom data is collected. In the last three years, 2,200 children have spent over 6 months in hospital; 245 of these children apparently spent more than five years in hospital.*
>
> *(DfES 2004a)*

So yet again, the specific needs of disabled children are not known.

Families can organize their own respite through a variety of non-social services providers including hospital units, residential community health units, private or voluntary schemes. Again, despite safeguards, these children are not under the protection of the review system. Cases have been known where a boarding school has been used to the maximum offered, and children have then been placed in more than one different health unit for holiday and weekend respite (Morris 1995:56) – all of which provision has been outside the Looked After system.

There is a risk that excessive use of these services, while providing relief and support to the family, will ultimately disadvantage children: a delicate balance. It is quite clear that systems to monitor the well-being of these children should be in place.

Looked After children

The previous section has drawn attention to the vulnerability of disabled children who live away from home but are not Looked After in the legal sense. We now come to children who are Looked After (both voluntarily and on legal orders) and who therefore do come under the provisions and protection of the Looked After children's review regulations. As stated above, these regulations form valuable safeguards which prevent children from drifting purposelessly around the care system, and should eventually ensure that each child has a permanent family: preferably supported at home within their birth family or, where that is not possible, in a permanent substitute family.

According to some definitions, over a quarter of all children in care are disabled (Gordon et al 2000). However, disability is the *principal reason* for becoming Looked After in only 4% of situations: about two-thirds of all children come into care because of abuse or neglect. Put another way, children are largely entering care for reasons other than disability, but many Looked After children are disabled (DCSF 2008).

Disabled children in temporary foster care

The first placement for many children entering the Looked After system is temporary care. Recent data show that 59 500 children were Looked After in England in March 2008, of whom 71% were living with foster carers. The total number of children in care rose gradually in the 10 years to 2004 and since then has fallen slightly. The percentage in foster care has increased (www.dfes.gov.uk). In 2005 there was an estimated shortfall of around 8000 foster families (DfES/National Statistics 2005) and it is believed this is still the case.

Research shows that 40% of the most severely and multiply disabled children are in foster care as opposed to 7% in residential establishments (Gordon et al 2000). However, Looked After disabled children are still generally less likely than other children to be placed with foster families: 21% of these children as opposed to 31% of non-disabled children. This is most regrettable.

In terms of 'outcomes', fostering research by Quinton (2004:92) has shown that 'special needs children did *better* on all the measures of outcome' than non-disabled children, and placements of children with physical disabilities were very unlikely to disrupt.

Disabled children in family-based short-break care
Children in social services short-break care for over 24 hours are classed as Looked After and their case must be reviewed through care planning. No single placement is to last for more than 4 weeks and the total duration of placements must not exceed 120 days in any 12-month period. For review purposes, a series of short-term placements may be treated as a single placement. While short breaks of this kind are a necessary support service for families, there have been some concerns that the child's view is not always canvassed. Again, a delicate balance must be struck if children are to be sustained with their families in the community.

There is also research to show that short-breaks schemes are less used than residential provision by Black and minority ethnic families. It has been argued that this is because of the necessity to negotiate directly with the carers, or because Black families fear that carers may not meet their child's cultural or religious needs (Flynn 2002:12).

Disabled children in residential care
The general issues for children who live away from home in residential settings were explored above. Disabled children who become Looked After are more likely than other children to be placed in residential care and thus, despite good practice, to be disadvantaged. According to Stuart and Baines (2004a) the vast majority of these children are White children (reflecting the profile of all Looked After children) between the ages of 10 and 15 – again, not a surprise. A government report says:

> *Because of the framework of reviews for looked after children there is less professional disquiet about this group of children, although there are concerns about the timeliness and quality of their reviews compared to their non-disabled peers who are looked after.*
>
> **(DfES 2004a)**

There are messages in this statement for all professionals who are invited to attend such reviews: although the safeguard of the review system is in place, a rigorous and objective scrutiny of the needs of the young person is clearly required.

Children who need 'permanence'
A minority of children who come into care do not return home, and research suggests that some of these children never achieve true 'permanence' through adoption or fostering. In fact, of 130 3–11 year-olds whose plan was adoption, fewer than two-thirds were still in adoptive families at follow-up, and 12% led very disrupted lives (Selwyn et al 2006). It is likely that some of these children are disabled. My own research, which

looked at children featured for permanence in BAAF's *Be My Parent* newspaper during one quarter of 2003, showed that 40% of the 350 children featured each month had some form of 'special need'; 20% had significant impairments and 5% had very serious impairments (Cousins 2006:5). Ivaldi's seminal research on children adopted from care (Ivaldi 2000) showed that prospective adopters are, in theory at least, wary of taking a disabled child, though when adoptions are examined, 40% of adopted children had at least one developmental difficulty, learning difficulty, medical problem or hereditary risk, and many had multiple difficulties. Disabled children are more likely to be placed for adoption with single carers (Owen 1999).

Many disabled children who need permanent new families are under 5 years old. Ivaldi (2000) shows that the most delay in family-finding generally is for boys over 2½ years who are to be adopted singly, and for Black and mixed parentage children. Disability adds a new dimension: children *under* 2½ with developmental difficulties (especially single boys again) wait a long time; and children with severe medical problems wait twice as long as others – particularly boys and children *over* 2½ years of age. One disturbing feature to emerge is that Black disabled children are more likely to be placed with White families.

Legal status
Many severely disabled children are Looked After on a voluntary basis under Section 20 of the Children Act 1989 rather than on legal orders. Here, parents who are unable to care for their child at home have full parental responsibility for decisions made in the care situation. Occasionally, parental requirements may not always be in tune with the child's best interests. In long-term planning, parents can veto permanence through adoption, or turn down specific prospective adopters whom social workers believe might be suitable. The child can thereby stay for an unacceptably long time in temporary care whilst awaiting a new permanent family.

Adoption by foster carers
There is evidence (Ivaldi 2000) that permanent (even adoptive) placements with foster carers are arising from these temporary arrangements. Attachments inevitably develop and carers see beyond the impairment to become fond of the child. Although there is a risk that the child may be continuing in a transracial placement, these 'matches' are in other respects thought to be robust. In December 2005 Special Guardianship was introduced which provides kinship carers and former foster carers (and others) with a new form of permanence somewhere between fostering and adoption.

Promoting and profiling children
According to Ivaldi (2000), only 13% of adopters said in advance hypothetically that they could take a child with a mental disability, 21% a physical disability, and 47% a medical condition whereas they seemed to be much less concerned about sexual and physical abuse. This is often a question of educating adopters and challenging the fears and prejudices that surround disability. The way in which disabled children are profiled and promoted is crucial (Cousins 2008). Workers must:

- avoid highlighting the impairment as if this were the only important feature;
- know the real child and check the child's view;
- portray the child vividly as an individual, without clichés;
- be honest, accurate, confidential and respectful;
- include aspects of daily living that the child can manage.

Profiles which stipulate 'type of family' – such as 'two-parent' or 'child must be the youngest' – immediately rule out some possible families. Prescribing the detail of contact arrangements or 'adoption only' can also be off-putting. Adoption support must be stressed – and delivered. If we do not get these basic issues right, some children will end up among those who will never have a family simply because we have erected spurious barriers at the start.

Conclusion

Most disabled children are cared for well in the community by their families. Even there, they are at risk of living in poverty, and of becoming marginalized by agencies and services. For the small number who live day to day elsewhere and for those who cannot return home permanently, their pathway is complex and risky. They are more likely to be placed in residential provision and to become chronically isolated from their families.

This most precious human right – the right to family life, upon which so much of children's future mental health rests, is often in jeopardy. This chapter has attempted to highlight the plight of these children so that readers from across the professional spectrum can be alert to their vulnerability.

It is recommended that all those who come into contact with disabled children should ask the following two fundamental questions.

- Does this child have a sense of home and family?
- Who is monitoring this child's long-term needs?

It is hoped that this chapter has provided the incentive to ask these questions and the ammunition to challenge unsatisfactory answers. Disabled children need families.

Chapter 2

Invisibility, Disability and the Problems of Public Care

Mary Mather

Introduction

The birth of a profoundly disabled child is an event that rocks any family to its foundations. It tests the bonds of relationships and the strengths of parents to the point of failure. Those families who manage to overcome this trauma and somehow keep going deserve the greatest respect because the level of support given to these families by society is often extremely poor. There are 49 000 severely disabled children in Britain. The great majority of them (91%) live at home imposing great strains on family life. Health and social services input to parents is not properly coordinated and 37% of families have been in contact with eight or more professionals (Heath and Smith 2004). Respite and residential care is scarce and difficult to obtain.

The number of severely disabled children in need of long-term care is set to increase as advances in medicine mean that more disabled children are surviving longer. However, compared with other children, children with a disability are more likely to live in poverty, have short-term breaks away from their families, use respite care, attend a residential school or ultimately become Looked After by local authorities.

- There are 61 100 children Looked After by local authorities in England, 64% on care orders, 35% by voluntary agreement.
- In 2004 the Department of Education and Skills estimated that approximately 2 400 children became Looked After primarily in response to a disability.

The number of children with a disability who have come into care for other reasons is unknown. In addition approximately 8 000 children per year receive an agreed series of short-term breaks and there are 2 800 unaccompanied asylum-seeking children, some of whom will be disabled (Department for Education and Skills (DfES)/National Statistics 2005). This is a large, invisible and uniquely deprived, population of children.

All children with disability suffer multiple disadvantages. Being Looked After by a local authority adds to this disadvantage. Looked After children with a disability suffer from the health problems experienced by all Looked After children but the added effect of their disability often compounds and intensifies their problems. Research into the outcomes for these children is very limited, their views and wishes are largely unknown and most importantly the failings of the system which initially brought them into care are largely unchallenged by society.

The health problems of all Looked After children
Children and young people who are Looked After are among the most socially excluded and unhealthy groups of children in the UK. Over the last 10 years, national and international research has indicated that these children have profoundly increased health needs in comparison with children and young people from comparable socioeconomic backgrounds.

A high percentage of Looked After children come into care with significant physical and mental health problems (Dimigen et al 1999, Skuse and Ward 1999, Skuse et al 2001). Fifty-two per cent have a physical condition that requires outpatient treatment (Skuse et al 2001). They also have high rates of mental health problems. In one study 45% of Looked After children between 5 and 17 years of age were assessed as having at least one psychiatric disorder (Meltzer et al 2003). Particularly high rates of self-harm and suicide are found in those living in secure accommodation (Richardson and Joughin 2000).

Unhealthy lifestyles are common in Looked After children. Compared with an equivalent non-care population, studies on Looked After children show higher levels of substance misuse; including cigarette smoking (Williams et al 2001, Meltzer et al 2003) and higher rates of teenage conceptions and early pregnancy (Corlyon and McGuire 1997). Immunization programmes are often incomplete (Hill et al 2003). Dental health is poor, few visit a dentist regularly and significantly more Looked After children need dental treatment (Williams et al 2001). At a time when childhood obesity and the diets of children are under increasing national scrutiny, virtually nothing is known about the nutritional status of Looked After children. For many however, contact with their social workers still means a trip to a fast food outlet and a meal high in calories, salt and saturated fats.

School failure also impacts on health. Educational achievements remain low with only 56% of young people sitting one GCSE compared with 96% of the general population. A higher percentage will be excluded from school (DfES/National Statistics 2004). A disrupted education then means that young people miss out on school-based health promotion and sexual health programmes.

The challenges faced by the health services in meeting the health needs of Looked After children are now well known. Preserving the family and medical history of Looked After children is difficult. Confidentiality and obtaining consent for treatments can be problematic (Mather et al 1997). The drawbacks of the isolated annual medical examination are now well recognized but the challenge of moving to long-term health assessment which actually improves health in a measurable way, remains to be met. Training in the particular health needs of minority ethnic groups remains woefully inadequate (Mather 2000). Standards and indicators for Looked After children still tend to focus on illness rather than health (Howell 2001).

In order to grow and develop children need long-term, consistent permanent relationships. No system of health care will ever overcome the effects of multiple moves. Whenever permanent placements are elusive health outcomes are always poor. Placement moves can further disrupt a child's health care and medical records may not always follow the child. Trying to provide good health care for children placed out of borough remains an elusive goal.

The views of Looked After children and young people without disability are now well known. They can be overwhelmed by stigma and low self-esteem. They resent being different from their peer group. They have other priorities in their lives and health care can seem relatively unimportant. They can often resent the annual health assessment carried out just because they are Looked After. There is often a real fear of physical examination and as they get older many refuse to attend. Being in care is such an all-enveloping feature of their lives that they may find it impossible to care about health or imagine life after care (Mather et al 1997).

A commitment to improving the physical health and emotional well-being of all Looked After children is high on both local and central government agendas. The ongoing dilemma for the UK is that Looked After children continue to have poor health outcomes and the NHS has still not been able to reverse their health inequalities. The dilemma for British social care is that despite a massive public investment of nearly £1 billion since 1998 in *Quality Protects* (England) (www.dcsf.gov.uk/qualityprotects/) and *Children First* (Wales) (www.childrenfirst.wales.gov.uk) plus a very high political profile, preserving normal childhood experiences and achieving good adult outcomes for Looked After children remains as elusive as ever.

Given this fairly bleak picture, how do Looked After children with a disability fare in this system? Before discussing the added disadvantage that disability brings, it is first necessary to describe the changing nature of childhood disability.

The changing face of disability in childhood

The straightforward assumptions of the past about disability in childhood are largely based on the presence of physical disability. Even the definition of disability in the 1989 Children Act has an almost biblical tone in the way disability is defined. In this most modern and far-reaching piece of legislation ever passed on British children, a child is defined as disabled if 'he is blind, deaf or dumb or suffers from mental disorder of any kind or is substantially and permanently handicapped by illness, injury or congenital deformity' (Children Act 1989).

There is a marked contrast between this simplistic language and the reality of daily life for parents and professionals coping with a disabled child today. For them, a disabled child will often have robust physical health but is very likely to have a problematic combination of severe learning disabilities[1] and very challenging behaviours. One study from Northern Ireland highlights this changing profile of childhood disability (McConkey et al 2004). The analysis of 108 children, all of whom had spent 90 days or more away from home in the preceding 12 months, was as follows:

- 10% had moderate learning disabilities;
- 51% had severe learning disabilities;
- 29% had profound learning disabilities.

Of the 108 children:

- 50% had challenging behaviour;
- 33% had severe communication problems;
- 20% had an autistic spectrum disorder;
- 14% were technologically dependent;
- only 10% of the children had a physical disability;
- there were no children with hearing or vision difficulties and none had a chronic illness;
- the median age of the children was 14 years suggesting that most families had struggled long and hard for many years before asking for help.

The increasing number of children diagnosed with autistic spectrum disorders represents a particular challenge. With better methods of assessments and diagnosis and a greater understanding of the behavioural and social problems which autistic children experience, there has been a marked increase in the numbers of children identified as having an autistic spectrum disorder. It can be very difficult to get the needs of this particular group recognized. Anyone who has ever tried to get an orange badge for a behaviourally challenging, yet very healthy autistic child can testify. Where parking is concerned, only impaired physical mobility counts with most local authorities. Parents who have to drag a terrified child, kicking and screaming to the shops are often patronizingly told that their child 'can walk' and 'buggies are not provided for restraint'.

Why children with disabilities come into public care

Until the 1970s, children with severe and profound learning disability were often accommodated in long-term hospitals, whilst those with severe hearing loss, visual impairment or chronic medical conditions like epilepsy were often educated in

---

1   North American usage: mental retardation.

residential boarding schools. Both forms of institutional care have now disappeared but have not been replaced by equivalent local services, which give parents a break from the demands of 24/7 care. There is a serious national shortage of both respite care and short breaks. This shortage has been compounded by an increase in the number of children surviving into their teenage years who are technologically dependent or have challenging behaviours.

In London in 2004, amidst widespread media coverage and national public sympathy for the parents, a High Court Judge, decided that an extremely disabled 10-month old baby should be allowed to die without any additional treatment when her condition deteriorated (England and Wales High Court Decisions 2004). Whatever the rights and wrongs of this decision, few commentators in the media furore that followed imagined what life could have been like for her parents if they had been able to take their baby home.

A severely disabled baby needs constant care, usually around the clock. This baby may have a high level of feeding problems, can cry inconsolably for hours or have frequent, frightening seizures. Even the most devoted parent can rapidly become exhausted and this exhaustion is made worse by a number of painful realizations. It begins to dawn on everyone that this problem is forever. Their child will have the needs of a baby for life and may never be able to live independently. Parents often have to face the stark choice of neglecting the needs of their other children in order to care for their baby. One parent, or possibly both, will have to give up work impoverishing and isolating the family. The relationship between the parents may not survive the lethal combination of exhaustion, poverty and constant anxiety. Disability often leads to separation or divorce when one parent simply cannot stand the strain and walks away. A child with a severe disability nearly always means a family that is equally disabled.

Under these unremitting pressures, a family needs a lot of help and support to survive. Yet despite our much-vaunted welfare state, such families get disgracefully little help.

There are 49 000 severely disabled children in Britain. The great majority (91%) live at home with their families (Heath and Smith 2004). Nearly half (48%) of their beleaguered and exhausted families receive no help whatsoever (Mencap 2001). There is a shocking mismatch between the vast sums spent on a baby in neonatal intensive care and the very small amount spent on the family after that baby goes home. According to government figures (2003) only 20% of families with a disabled relative get any short breaks and 34% of families are receiving fewer services than they were in the previous year (Department of Health (DH) 2003).

On average in the UK, 6 children out of every 1000 births are born with a severe or profound learning disability. With about 800 000 live births per year, this means that 4 800 babies are born each year with severe or profound learning difficulty. This represents about 90 babies a week (Heath and Smith 2004). It is however very hard to assess the numbers of disabled individuals in Britain because, despite an obligation to keep a register of disabled people in order to better provide long-term planning, few local authorities or other bodies have complied with this regulation.

Under the current system, disabled children and their families are entitled to an assessment of their needs by their local authority. Social workers should visit any family with a child with a severe disability to assess the home and the family's needs. The family should then be allocated support in terms of a certain number of hours of domiciliary care, respite care, equipment or structural modifications to their home. This allocation is however subject to budgetary restrictions and the availability of appropriately trained staff. Despite the individual nature of these assessments, most of the resulting care plans are, at the end of the day, very similar. This is because there is only a limited choice of services and it is the amount, rather than the type of service provided that changes. In 2003, in a study of 76 families caring for a profoundly disabled child:

- only 60% had had a care assessment;
- only 20% had been allocated a short break;
- unsurprisingly, 80% had reached breaking point (Mencap 2003).

The National Service Framework for Children (DH 2004a) aims to ensure that disabled children 'enjoy the highest quality of life possible' and 'their needs and those of their families are promptly and sensitively addressed'. Yet behind closed doors some of our most vulnerable children are being denied their basic human rights. Whilst millions are being spent on providing disabled access to public buildings, thousands of disabled children are unable to safely access their own home.

Box 2.1 Jack

Jack was diagnosed with Duchenne muscular dystrophy when he was 3 years old. When he was 6, in order to meet his future care needs, his family moved into a bungalow, which his parents are still buying on a mortgage. By the time Jack was 9 years old, his parents needed to adapt their property in order to allow wheelchair access to all the rooms on the ground floor. The local council assessed Jack's family as being able to pay for these alterations themselves. Jack's mother does not work because she has to care for him full time. His father's limited income will not support the additional mortgage repayments. Jack is now 10 and although he uses a wheelchair at school, he cannot get it into his own home. Here his mother and father physically carry him from room to room.

Families with disabled children do not have the right to money to make their homes accessible and there is only limited help available through grants. Parents are means tested for any structural adaptations to their home. A standard bedroom and bathroom ground floor extension costs in the region of £50 000. As Jack becomes heavier, and his parents become older it is only a matter of time before they are unable to cope and make a request for Jack to have respite care or even to be accommodated.

Many parents of disabled children eventually give up after a long struggle to cope, totally exhausted and feeling desperately guilty. In a study in Northern Ireland 33% of children came into care because their parents were not coping compared with 18% who had experienced neglect or suspected abuse. Parental profiles spoke volumes about the family struggles that had preceded their children's entry into public care:

- 15% lived with a single parent;
- 12% of the families in this study had two or more disabled children;
- in 14%, the mother or father had a physical health problem;
- in 12% the parents had mental health problems;
- 8% of parents suffered from drug or alcohol misuse;
- 8% of parents had learning disabilities (McConkey et al 2004).

The ethical problems of Looked After children with disabilities

Once a child becomes Looked After, putting the welfare of the child at the centre of professional practice can be very difficult. The rest of this chapter will focus on the unique ethical problems that can arise in the day to day management of these vulnerable children.

Providing continuing high-quality health care

The delivery of health care in the NHS is still largely dependent upon a child and family living at a relatively stable address, establishing a relationship with a local general practitioner who in turn, has a relationship with the local hospital and mental health services.

Foster carers for children with disability are always in very short supply. A child with a disability is therefore much more likely to be placed with an agency carer out of district. When this happens, the health care of the child will then transfer to a new team of general practitioners, paediatricians and therapists who will need time to get to know the child. Health services always take time to set up in a new district. There may be long local waiting lists for physiotherapy and speech therapy services. Medical records take time to arrive. At the same time the child may also have had to move schools. It is often forgotten, in the desperate search to find at suitable placement, that multiple moves are traumatizing for any child. In the child with profound disability, this trauma can present as deteriorating behaviour.

Significant numbers of disabled Looked After children will eventually be placed in residential schools, many in 52-week placements. These children will inevitably lose total contact with the local health services that knew them well. In residential schools, health care is often provided by a visiting general practitioner with a contract to visit the school on a termly basis supported by a local out of hours general practitioner cooperative that provides emergency care.

Since staff are understandably reluctant to take responsibility for caring overnight for a child within a residential unit, disabled children with acute medical problems such as chest infections or seizures are inevitably admitted to the local hospital as an emergency. Long waits in the accident and emergency department and overnight admissions to a paediatric ward are very common. The child will then be cared for by hospital staff that have never met the child. Doctors, who are not able to speak to parents, cannot obtain a comprehensive medical history and have no access to medical records. The care worker who takes the child to hospital will often have to return to the unit leaving the child alone with strangers.

This intermittent, impersonal health care is totally inadequate for a child with profound disabilities and cannot compare with that provided by a caring parent. All parents monitor their child on a daily basis, recognize even minor changes in that child's heath status, take responsibility for care during an acute illness and rarely leave their child alone if a hospital admission is necessary. Sadly the inverse care law still applies to the disabled Looked After child, those in most need of good care are the least likely to obtain it.

Stopping treatment
Stopping active treatment and palliative care can be an emotional, legal and ethical minefield. Many disabled children whose parents receive respite care are not recognized as either 'accommodated' or 'Looked After' under the Children Act. This means that care plans and reviews are often not carried out as legislation requires. Some disabled children are spending time away from home in short-term placements, particularly hospitals and hospices, without any knowledge or involvement of social services. Many 'drift' into public care with an uncertain legal status but are still likely to lose contact with their families. In this legal limbo, valid consent can be very problematic to obtain.

Box 2.2 Amil

Amil is nearly 3 and voluntarily accommodated. He was born with an extensive structural brain abnormality. He has microcephaly (a small head), poorly controlled epilepsy, cerebral palsy and severe learning disabilities. He is probably blind. The congenital abnormality in his brain involves his brain stem and Amil cannot maintain his fluid balance, his blood pressure or his plasma cortisol. He has increasingly recurrent episodes when he stops breathing and has been resuscitated three times. Amil's mother was 14 when he was born. She was brought up in care and cannot cope with the complexities of her son's medical needs.

The consultant paediatrician caring for Amil and his foster carer believe that he has not only a very limited life expectancy, but that his quality of life is poor. They do not believe that any further active resuscitation is in his best interests if he stops breathing again. His young mother is understandably ambivalent and bewildered and wants 'the doctors to do everything they can'. His social worker is unable to make a decision and the local authority is instructing a barrister. The decision whether or not to resuscitate Amil will be fought out in court. The costs of the subsequent legal action will seriously deplete the local authority budget and reduce services for other disabled children.

Although this may be the right course of action in such a difficult case as Amil's, it would rarely happen to a child living at home with its parents. In most cases, these sensitive decisions can be made in private, over time, between parents and doctors as a child's condition slowly worsens. The parents will be supported in making the decision that they think is right for their child and professionals will respect the difficult choices they have faced in coming to a final conclusion.

When birth parents have not been directly caring for their child for many years, who is the best judge of what course of action is in that child's best interest? It is often the foster carer, teacher, nurse or therapist working with the child on a daily basis who has the most insight into that child's quality of life. However, in any court process, the opinion of the most involved individuals is rarely sought. In a legal decision-making forum, the people who will be primarily consulted will be the child's parents, then his social worker and then the medical expert who often only sees the child every 6 months. The opinion of the foster carer may only be sought as a last resort but will carry no legal weight. The opinion of a child's teachers, therapists and day to day helpers is rarely, if ever, considered.

Starting treatment and obtaining consent
Disabled children with less complex problems than Amil may also require other types of medical intervention. Who gives consent when a disabled Looked After child requires an investigation involving an anaesthetic, such as magnetic resonance imaging or when consent is needed for surgery or drug therapy or gastrostomy feeding? These decisions can be just as difficult as the more serious question of palliative care and the stopping of active medical treatment. Consent for medical treatment is often delegated to the director or assistant director of social services, who has never met the child. How in these circumstances can consent be fully informed?

Drug treatment

Drug treatment is a particularly controversial area. Many of the disabled children in the care system have little or no speech. They do not have access to signing systems and can have complex challenging behaviour. The use of powerful antipsychotic drugs is progressively increasing in this population of children. Ideally medication should only be used to improve the quality of a child's life, to help a child learn or to treat medical conditions such as epilepsy. There is however no doubt that reducing challenging behaviours also reduces high staffing levels and therefore placement costs. Drugs like methylphenidate (Ritalin®, Concerta®), which reduce hyperactivity, can also help to prevent placement breakdown.

- Who decides when a drug is being used largely as a chemical restraint?
- Who is the best person to make the decision to start medication?
- Who should then consent to treatment?
- Who should monitor the effects of medication and who should decide when it is no longer necessary?

The long-term monitoring of medication is then often made more difficult because the child with challenging behaviours is more likely to have a placement disruption when the monitoring of the treatment then transfers to a new team of doctors.

Child protection
Children living away from home are uniquely vulnerable to abuse. A number of small studies have suggested that the prevalence of abuse in the disabled population is actually greater than it is in the general population. All children, whatever the underlying disability, will become worse and their behaviour will deteriorate if they are abused or their needs neglected. When behaviour problems worsen in the Looked After child, there is a tendency to attribute any behaviour deterioration to the underlying disorder. Child protection issues in this population of children are difficult to address and resolve. There are no national statistics about the incidence of abuse in disabled Looked After children.

Children with complex difficulties are vulnerable on many fronts. Disabled children, like all children, have an overwhelming need for affection and friendship that can be exploited by manipulative abusers. Many are isolated, totally dependent and inexperienced. They have never been taught the norms of adult behaviour. These children can be deprived of sex education and training in assertiveness. A child's low self-image, compounded by the trauma of rejection by their families and multiple moves, discourages disclosure.

The notion of personal privacy is meaningless for the severely disabled. They have an age inappropriate dependency and are totally reliant on others for personal care, dressing and toileting. If a child has a physical disability it is impossible for them to escape from the presence of an abuser who may be responsible for their intimate care, carried out behind closed doors. During a 24-hour shift in a residential unit, the staff will change several times. There is, in addition, a constant turnover of staff, as the work is poorly paid and the hours are unsocial. Consequently numerous people can enter and leave the life of a child in a short period of time. Care workers, drivers, escorts, therapists, social workers often change with bewildering speed. The more people there are in a child's life the greater the risk that screening policies, designed to detect abusers, will fail. There is sometimes a very naive view that children with disabilities are 'immune' to abuse whereas their vulnerability, powerlessness, lack of assertiveness and difficulties in communication may well make them 'attractive' to the abuser.

Many Looked After children in public care have problems with communication. A significant percentage will be completely non-verbal. At an even more basic level, children with disability are frequently not even given the language to disclose abuse because they are not taught what are perceived to be unpleasant or sexually explicit words. Very few professionals have the skill to communicate with a child who is reliant solely on non-verbal means of communication. The usual methods of interviewing children do not work and criminal proceedings are rare because of the inadmissibility of most evidence.

Total denial by the abuser and disbelief by the carer may precipitate severely challenging behaviour, which is then seen as more 'evidence' of a child's unreliability as a witness.

There needs to be a very high level of awareness of the risks of abuse by both professionals and parents. All professionals need to recognize that:

- disabled children and adults have normal emotional and sexual needs;
- all children need sex education and training in assertiveness;
- tools need to be found to give children the language to disclose;
- more skilled child protection professionals are needed to work directly with children with disability.

There also needs to be a greater awareness and training on the part of the law to ensure that the welfare of the child is protected, even if the evidential base for criminal proceedings is weak.

Talking to children who cannot talk
Putting the interests of children first, means that all who try to work with them have an obligation to find out about their wishes and feelings. Over half of disabled children in contact with social services have little or no speech. However, few professionals working with them have the specialist training to communicate with them. It is very rare for social workers to have any training in specialist communication even when those social workers are from Children with Disabilities Teams and are carrying caseloads where large numbers of children have no speech (see Chapter 9).

The Who? Cares Trust Report *Still Missing* looked at 66 cases presented to a London Resource Panel (Morris, 1995). In 54 of these cases no attempt had been made to ascertain the child's view. In at least five cases the social worker had not even seen the child. Typically the section of the form headed 'Child's view' was left blank. The social worker had made comments such as 'she is unable to verbally communicate and therefore her view is not available', or 'It is not possible to know what his views are owing to his level of disability'. There were a number of occasions when the child was already spending time in a residential unit, but in only one instance did the social worker observe him there to find out whether he was happy. Only 27% of the caseload of one city council's Children with Disabilities Team used speech to communicate, and another 25% had limited speech.

The report then analysed similar cases presented to a Country Resource Panel. Of the 24 cases submitted, in 11 instances the social worker had written 'Not applicable' in the section headed 'Child's perception of needs' and in another 11 cases the section was left completely blank. The same report points out how rare it is for children to be observed by social workers in residential units and how common it is for the social workers to speak solely with staff because 'the child cannot make their needs known'.

The parents of children with disability who know their children well can often read their facial expressions, gestures, vocalizations and body language accurately. Many have taught themselves signing systems or have computer-aided communication systems. This situation is rarely replicated when children are Looked After and these failures need addressing with urgency. There is currently little evidence that disabled children's wishes and feelings about their placement are being ascertained, that their feelings of grief and rejection are being considered and addressed and that they are being involved in important decisions about their lives.

Supporting foster carers
The status of foster carers within local authorities is sometimes ambiguous and often peripheral. They are neither members of staff nor outsiders and they have a low status within the organization. Most foster carers come into fostering because they are motivated by a wish to do something for children in need. They expect the local authority fostering service to have a similar commitment. Preparation before placement, training courses and foster care manuals usually lead carers to expect support in the form of visits, availability, teamwork, problem solving and responsiveness to crises throughout the 24 hours of the day. If a foster carer is caring for a profoundly disabled child, the availability of this support is even more important.

There is sometimes a mindset within social services departments that treats disabled and Looked After children as if these children represent two mutually exclusive categories. Often different teams deal with these children. In a large study of foster care, many commented on the increasing demands of their time from having to attend meetings and reviews, visits to schools and doctors, keeping records, working with parents and promoting contact while confronting constant fears about false allegations of abuse. Reasons why even the most dedicated foster carers will stop caring for a disabled child include:

● infrequent social work visits;
● cancelled visits;
● unavailability;
● unresponsiveness and lack of local authority support (Triseloitis et al 1999).

Paradoxically, a child's foster carer is often the one person in the complex network of professionals surrounding the child who has the most insight into that child's needs and the most expertise in dealing with a child's difficulties on a day to day basis. It is frequently the foster carer who:

● takes the child to hospital;
● is directly responsible for the child's health care whilst not being able to consent to the treatment or medication suggested;
● carries out most physiotherapy and occupational therapy programmes supported by a very occasional professional review;
● liases with the child's school and supports school-based programmes.

Foster carers for children with severe disabilities are difficult to identify and the demand always exceeds supply. Most professionals can however testify to the dramatic and unexpected improvements that even the most severely disabled children have made in the right foster or adoptive family. Impersonal residential units are not the right place for the most vulnerable children in our society and need to be seen as very much a last resort. More support to the beleaguered fostering service seems to be one of the best ways to prevent more Looked After children going down this road.

The future

When children with a disability enter the care system, it is largely because their parents have been increasingly unable to cope with the burdens of caring for them. A Mencap survey (2001) found:

- 60% of parents spent more than 10 hours per day on basic care, with one-third of this group providing 24-hour continuous care;
- 57% were spending more than 8 hours per day on therapy and education;
- on average parents were woken three times every night (Mencap 2001).

The long-stay hospitals of the 1970s and the 1980s have been closed down and have not been replaced by alternative provision or even an equivalent amount of respite care or short breaks.

The lack of short-term breaks to relieve family stress and prevent family breakdown is a national scandal. There is an urgent need for more preventative services in the community for disabled children and a particular need for services that can deal effectively with challenging behaviour. There is also an urgent need to find better ways of communicating with disabled children to prevent their behaviour deteriorating as a result of frustration and unrelieved distress. There is a need for advocacy for this most vulnerable group of children and a pressing need to find ways of identifying the views of the children themselves who are so often powerless in what is happening around them. A lack of essential basic data prevents proper planning and there is an urgent need for greater monitoring.

Families living with a disabled child tend to know what they need. They would much rather choose care services themselves rather than receive insufficient help from local authorities. Unfortunately the rigidity of the current system does not give families any personal choice. Out of the £540 million spent by social services on disabled children, £140 million (26%) is spent on assessment and commissioning whilst services to support families become more stretched and fewer in both quantity and quality (Heath and Smith 2004). If fewer children with disabilities are to spend their lives Looked After by social services then the system, which supports them and their families whilst they are at home, is in urgent need of reform.

Chapter 3

Disabled Children Living Away from Home in the Care System: Coordinating medical and health services

Heather Payne

Introduction

Children and young people in the public care (Looked After children) represent about half a percent of the child population in England (British Association for Adoption and Fostering 2007). Being Looked After[1] is an administrative category that contains a heterogeneous group of children and young people, ranging from birth to adolescence, from fully able to severely disabled, with a variable amount of placement security and stability. There will be a great variety of patterns of contact with their family of origin, and the child may be located in a wide range of settings, living with family and friends under a care order, in shared care, foster care or residential placement. Looked After children are a population group at greater risk than the average child of:

- physical disability (DfES 2004b);
- mental illness and disorders (McCann et al 1996);
- as well as the long-term effects of abuse, neglect and social disadvantage.

Children with a disability are, similarly, a heterogeneous group. They may present at any age from birth to adolescence, with a wide range of conditions and problems that may affect their physical, emotional, intellectual or social development. Children with a disability are also much more vulnerable to abuse (Carlile 2002) as a result of immobility, or limited ability or communication.

---

1 For definitions of Looked After and Disability see Chapter 1.

> **Box 3.1 Clinical vignettes to illustrate the wide range of need:**
>
> - a boy of 3 with cerebral palsy with four limb involvement and cortical blindness requiring help with mobility, communication, feeding, toileting and sensory augmentation;
> - a young man of 15 with Duchenne muscular dystrophy requiring help with mobility and assisted ventilation at night;
> - a boy of 12 with learning difficulties and autistic spectrum disorder;
> - a girl of 13 with attention-deficit–hyperactivity disorder (ADHD), and severe scarring to the lower body and genitalia following a non-accidental scald as a baby.

Whatever the needs of the child for health or medical and social care and education, it is important to focus on the rights of the child. Vulnerable groups share the problems of living at higher risk of poverty and deprivation, being marginalized and 'politically invisible' because of their lack of economic power or advocacy, and having difficulty in accessing services (the 'inverse care law' (Tudor Hart 1971), where those most in need of services are least able to access them.). Both Looked After and disabled children are more likely to come from an ethnic minority, and to miss out on services (Huang et al 2005).

Children who are Looked After or disabled are – first and foremost – children with all the rights, needs, demands and aspirations of all children and young people (www.unicef.org.uk/tz/rights/convention.asp). Meeting the child's needs requires moving away from a narrow biomedical focus towards interagency working that is child centred, building on the strengths of the families and the communities in which they live

Types of disability

Children with disability may be considered in the following classification for the purposes of exploring the evidence base (Sibert et al 2002). Categories for consideration are children:

- with physical disability and mobility problems;
- with sensory impairment (vision, hearing and speech and language impairment);
- with mental health problems, disorders or illness (depression, anxiety, ADHD, attachment problems, emotional and behavioural disorders);
- with learning disability including autism spectrum disorder and learning difficulties;
- requiring long-term ventilation;
- with long-term medical problems or life-limiting conditions;
- requiring burns and plastic surgery for congenital abnormalities;
- with head or spinal injuries requiring orthopaedic surgery and rehabilitation.

In reality, the situation for any individual child is often much more complicated, some children having high levels of comorbidity or multiple disabilities. The same principles of careful individual assessment apply even more strongly in these situations. Other groups of children and young people are also particularly vulnerable to the effects of the inverse care law. There are particular needs for services appropriate for adolescents (Fleming et al 2005) and the transition to adult services.

Disabled children entering the Looked After system

This happens for a range of different reasons. The following are the main reasons for a disabled child or sibling group to be Looked After by the local authority (Children Act 1989, Section 20 (accommodation) and Section 32 (care orders)).

- Placement in a foster home following abuse or neglect, (especially following shaken baby syndrome and subdural haemorrhage) for a short term (months) whilst assessment and long-term plans are completed.

- In a foster home following abuse or neglect and the failure of a rehabilitation plan to return the child to safety within the original family, leading to the need for a long-term placement.

- In a foster home, awaiting an adoptive home following relinquishment by birth family, due to the severity or nature of the child's disability.

- At home with the birth family, with visits to a foster home or residential unit as a planned long-term shared or respite care arrangement. This allows the disabled child to experience wider social contacts and gives their carers time for other children in the family.

- In a residential placement. This may be a special residential unit, hospital or hospice for children with severe physical illness or disability; a special school (e.g. for children with visual or hearing impairment, language disorders, autistic spectrum disorder); a children's home for older young people whose needs are not compatible with living in a foster family; or a secure unit for young people who are offending or self-harming.

In all situations where a child is both disabled and Looked After, the same principles of care apply:

- the child is a child first and foremost, not just disabled or Looked After;
- the child must have their overall best interests identified by a holistic and multidisciplinary approach;
- the child's wishes and feelings must be taken into account;
- all work should be in partnership with the child, their parents and carers.

Needs of children and services required

Both disabled children and Looked After children are identified as groups of Children in Need by the Children Act 1989, in that they need extra services to ensure their health and development. Being either disabled or Looked After is a marker for deprivation and poverty. The aim of the *Quality Protects* (www.dcsf.gov.uk/qualityprotects) and *Children First* (www.childrenfirst.wales.gov.uk) programmes in England and Wales respectively (which commenced in 1999) is to improve outcomes and life chances for all Children in Need.

A literature review on children with special health needs conducted in 2002 (Sibert et al concluded that the evidence base supporting the care of children who are disabled or Looked After is very sparse and very patchy. There are very few randomized controlled trials outside specific drug treatment such as methylphenidate for ADHD or botulinum toxin in cerebral palsy. There are also some effective cognitive behavioural interventions in child and adolescent mental health, but these are limited to short-term interventions (Wolpert 2002). In the absence of a robust evidence base, professional consensus and practice wisdom is the best available evidence. The involvement and inclusion of disabled and Looked After young people in shaping health services is an important theme for all future development.

The pattern of health care needs of children with disabilities has changed greatly over the past decades, and will continue to change. This includes factors such as:

● the better survival of very small babies, many with long-term difficulties like cerebral palsy;
● the reduced incidence of spina bifida;
● increased identification of specific learning difficulties, developmental coordination disorders and autistic spectrum disorder;
● complex special needs and more available treatments (such as intermittent ventilation, home oxygen, hospital at home, gastrostomy feeding, hospice beds)
● the specific needs of individual ethnic groups in a multicultural society, especially regarding language and communication;
● the wishes of parents and carers to become skilled and directly involved in caring for children and the professional support required to facilitate this (including information resources and evidence-based guidelines);
● the need for a smooth, planned transition for paediatric to adult services for adolescents and young people with ongoing health needs;
● appropriate training and support for the professionals working in multiprofessional teams to meet the needs of children and their families and carers (Abbott et al 2005).

Specific issues relevant to children who are Looked After
● A wide variation in the level and specificity of health services for Looked After children in different regions in the UK. This makes it extremely difficult to compare service outcomes or ensure equity of access to services for Looked After children. Children placed distant from their placing authority are particularly poorly served, as it becomes much more difficult for interprofessional working to take place.

- Children and young people in residential, secure accommodation and prison are an especially vulnerable group (Bundkl 2001). The rate of mental illness and mental health disorder is exceptionally high, young people may be placed far distant from home and family, with no oversight or coordination of health services.

Measuring performance baselines

If the aim is to achieve better health care and health outcomes for disabled Looked After children as a population, it is first necessary to identify and examine baseline measures of structure, process and outcome. In the absence of data specific to disabled Looked After children, it is possible to adduce evidence from general contexts and apply it as a desirable standard of care.

- Early diagnosis of disorders is desirable but there is little evidence for the use of screening programmes, except for universal neonatal hearing screen, hypothyroidism and phenylketonuria. The model of surveillance needed for all children should be as described in *Health for all Children* (Hall and Elliman 2003), responsive to the concerns of parents or carers and screening of high-risk groups (such as for mental health problems in Looked After children)

- Routine health care services should be available and accessible to all children, including primary medical and dental care (A general practitioner and dentist) and optician services. Community dental services often provide primary dental care for children who cannot access a general dental practitioner (Waldman and Perlman 2004).

- The disclosure of diagnosis and ongoing provision of information to parents and carers is recognized as being vital in maintaining support and empowerment for the primary carers of the child with a disability. This task is even more complex in the Looked After child, as the communication of information to all parties can be considerably more difficult in a logistical sense. The use of a Personal Child Health record that travels with the child, and is used by professionals and carers to share information, is a widely accepted model of good practice. Supporting parents and carers in searching for helpful information on the internet is also valuable.

- Coordination of care by a keyworker (where the child requires two or more separate professional inputs) is evidenced as valuable in improving quality of life for the child and carers. It is effective to promote the coordination of multiprofessional working at the level of the child and responsive to their needs.

- Coordination of multiagency working using shared criteria and databases (a disability register) is desirable. Unless agencies share information in a meaningful way, and use it as a basis for audit and quality improvement, there is unlikely to be improved joint working. Service boundaries are irrelevant to the child, and burdensome for parents and carers. For example, a child needing daily health care intervention during the school day must be enabled to receive it in school, rather than attend health premises for it.

- Clinical care pathways and managed clinical networks are effective in managing services for hearing impairment in children. They promote best practice and equity of service, offering maximal effectiveness and efficiency of service. They need central support, protected clinician time and adequate information technology resources

- Access to therapy services and equipment are a common problem for all children with a disability. The effective use of therapy time by focusing on assessment and planning a home programme of therapy allows efficient use of therapist time, and involvement of parents, cares and school in the intervention programme.

The health assessment process for Looked After children

Previous research has identified that Looked After children are at greater than average risk of health and developmental problems (Williams et al 2001). There is a statutory requirement (Children Act 1989) for a yearly Looked After Child health assessment process, requiring the child's needs to be assessed and a health care plan formulated. Historically, this was conducted as a medical examination. However, this is an excessively medically modelled approach, which does not offer appropriate support for health promotion, ascertaining the wishes and feeling of the child, promoting mental health or empowering young people and carers. A more appropriate model of care is now in widespread use in the UK, and uses a health assessment process delivered by nurses working within a multidisciplinary health team to identify and meet health needs (Wright 2004). Such a system is a 'best fit' of child need and service delivery, and is much more acceptable to Looked After children and young people of all ages.

The health assessment must lead to the formulation of a health care plan. This document should identify all the health problems and issues affecting the disabled Looked After child, and must contain a health action plan. The health care plan should address the identified health needs of the child (including mental health), and identify the actions to be taken, who should take them and by when.

Where disabled Looked After children have a diagnosed medical condition for which there is an established clinical care pathway or quality standard (e.g. asthma, long-term ventilation), the health care plan must incorporate it to ensure optimal management according to good clinical governance (DH 2004a).

A health record which travels with the Looked After child should be made available (Payne and Bulter 1998) and the plan should be communicated, subject to the consent of the child, to the parents, carers, social worker and primary care team (general practitioner) and, if relevant, education and keyworker.

Health promotion services should be offered (Hill and Watkins 2003) to all disabled Looked After children, both directly, and indirectly, to households where they live. Parents and carers should be offered education in healthy choices regarding diet, exercise, avoidance of smoking and drugs, safer sex and responsible use of alcohol.

Service coordination and quality

Effective coordination of all services which influence health for Looked After children should be monitored for each local authority area by a multiagency group which reports back to chief executive officers of health, social services and education as well as elected members. This would be an effective way of guarding against institutional abuse of Looked After children.

The use of managed clinical networks (www.wales.nhs.uk/sites/page.cfm?orgid=355 &pid=4560) for the coordination of health care for disabled Looked After children should be developed as a model which would allow local and regional comparisons of performance. This requires the collection of an agreed minimum data set and comparison within and between services and agencies, with systematic collection of health data, allowing proper scientific quality comparisons to be made. There should be agreed interagency protocols which are audited regularly. Views of service users (children, parents and carers) should be routinely sought (www.voicesfromcarecymru. org.uk/main.htm).

Appropriately trained and skilled secondary child health services need to be available to disabled Looked After children on an equitable basis. Each trust should ensure they have medical and nursing staff appropriately qualified and experienced in working with disability and Looked After children with appropriate time resources to see children and coordinate services. In particular, access to Child and Adolescent Mental Health services (CAMHS) is essential, to provide diagnostic and therapeutic work including post-abuse therapy and support.

Appropriately trained and skilled services from a range of other health professionals are required, particularly speech and language therapy and occupational therapy and an information support officer to coordinate and channel information to disabled Looked After children, their parents and carers

Children living outside their local health area, especially those in residential, secure or youth justice placements, are a subset of the most vulnerable Looked After children. They are very much more likely to have mental illness or disorder, and a specific need for health, social care and educational coordination. At present, these needs are unlikely to be met (Gould and Payne 2004).

Support for promoting mental health

A range of non-medical services are important for disabled Looked After children to ensure they have 'normalizing' experiences, including access to schooling and leisure activities. This can promote resilience (Rutter 1999) and is thus a valuable tool in promoting the overall physical and mental well-being of the child.

Respite care provision is an important issue for many carers (Johnson and Kastner 2005). There is frequently an inadequate supply of both quantity and type of care available. Respite carers caring for children who require any invasive procedures must be trained in performing that procedure (e.g. gastrostomy feeding, administering rectal valium, stoma care) on that specific child. This is a general requirement of insurance policies. The relevant health professionals (e.g. ward outreach nurses) must be engaged in supporting this training for carers as well as for parents.

Child protection systems should always be robustly in place. This should cover the continuum of child care needs, for the protection of the individual child and for the approval process for carers. The recommendations of the Protection of Children Act in performing Criminal Records Bureau checks, and taking up references, must be implemented for all carers. The system must be overseen by professionals who understand child protection needs and the vulnerability of disabled Looked After children.

A systematic assessment of educational needs for disabled Looked After children is important. There is a high prevalence of learning problems and language disorders among this group of children. If children are excluded from school, this can put intolerable pressures on a home placement and destroy placement stability (Stanley et al 2005). Such problems require prompt active management, with help to reintegrate to the school environment with the appropriate supports needed to maintain attendance.

Conclusions

- There is very little research evidence for planning effective health interventions for disabled Looked After children. This is a vulnerable population of uniquely deprived children and young people.
- The process of health assessment, health care delivery and coordination is acceptable and effective when based on a nurse specialist working as part of a multiprofessional health team for Looked After children (see Chapter 4).
- Coordinated information and planning systems are needed, and data should be collected to benchmark health service structure, process and outcome.
- Multidisciplinary working demands the setting up of properly resourced and coordinated teams with identified lead professionals for Looked After children including paediatrics, nursing, CAMHS, social services and education. The use of managed clinical networks and clinical care pathways for complex medical problems is likely to be beneficial.
- Health care of children placed out of health area, and all children in secure or youth justice placements, must be monitored as identifiable groups of the most vulnerable and needy children in our society.

Chapter 4

Health Promotion and Health Assessments for Looked After Children: The role of the clinical nurse specialist for Looked After children

Maraline Jones

Background and principles of practice

Clinical nurse specialists for Looked After children were established in the Borough of Caerphilly, Wales in 2000. Since then our work has evolved in keeping with service needs, child care legislation and the findings of evidence-based practice. This chapter describes the area where we work, the principles of practice, our arrangements with social services regarding health assessments for Looked After children and the current role of the clinical nurse specialists.

The Borough of Caerphilly was created in 1996 because of reorganisation of the local Gwent Unitary Authority. It is located on the western edge of Gwent and occupies 28 000 hectares with a population of 177 000. It is the largest unitary authority in Wales. Caerphilly stretches 40 km (23 miles) from north to south. In 2003 there were 4140 Looked After children in Wales, 350 in Caerphilly at any one time with more than 400 going through the Looked After system annually.

At the outset it was agreed that the service provided by the clinical nurse specialist for Looked After children would be child centred, evidence based (wherever possible) and have strong links with other professionals and families/carers involved with Looked After children. Professional groups we have established good working relationships with include:

- social services – the family placement team, the caseworkers/social workers for the children, the leaving care social workers, adoption support team and children services managers;
- the education department, including inclusion services;
- sexual health workers, drug and alcohol services, and youth outreach workers;
- child and adolescent mental health services (CAMHS), psychiatry, psychology, primary mental health team;
- generic primary health services for example health visitors and school nurses, paediatric and practice nurses;
- professionals allied to medicine, e.g. audiology, speech therapy, occupational therapy, physiotherapy, dietetics;
- professionals in the youth offending team;
- the children's rights officer;
- professionals in the children's disability team.

The health assessment

The Welsh Assembly Government issued guidance under section 25(8), 27(4), 28(4), of The Children Act 2004, and Section 7 of the Local Authority Social Services Act 1970 (Welsh Assembly Government (2007) *Towards a Stable Life and A Brighter Future*) Statutory Instrument 2007 No.307 (W26) schedule 7.-1:

> *The responsible authority must, in respect of each child who continues to be looked after or provided with accommodation by them, make arrangements for a registered medical practitioner or a registered nurse, to conduct an assessment, which may include a physical examination, of the child's state of health –*
>
> *at least once, and more frequently if the child's welfare requires it, in every period of six months before the child's fifth birthday; and*
>
> *at least once, and more frequently if the child's welfare requires it, in every period of twelve months after the child's fifth birthday.*
> **(Welsh Assembly Government 2007)**

There are two clinical nurse specialists in Caerphilly we undertake both the initial health assessments and the health assessment reviews for Looked After children from birth to leaving care. We also have links with the leaving care team and remain involved if the young person wants us to after they have left the care system. We work as part of a team for Looked After children with a consultant paediatrician and clerical support.

A study in South Wales, carried out in the late 1990s, of health assessments for Looked After children by medical officers or general practitioners found a poor uptake rate (11–51%) (Butler and Payne 1997). By contrast a pilot study involving clinical nurse specialists who delivered a service in the same area in 2000 had an uptake rate of 86%. It was therefore decided that all health assessments for Looked After children in Caerphilly would be carried out by clinical nurse specialists with a consultant paediatrician taking overall clinical responsibility until the change in the regulations mentioned above when nurses were given this responsibility in 2004. Clinical nurse specialists undertake both the initial and the review health assessments. If the health assessment raises medical or developmental worries the case is discussed with the consultant paediatrician who sees the child promptly when needed.

Over the past 8 years the clinical nurse specialists service has been shown to be efficient and safe. Children have told us that they did not want to see a doctor because they were not ill. They also told us that it was easier to talk to a nurse than to a doctor. A study by Jane Dove (Dove 2004, unpublished) has confirmed that children prefer a nurse-led service. The uptake for Looked After health assessments is now usually over 90% for the children living in the Caerphilly area.

Looked After children who are placed outside the local authority area
The Placement of Children (Wales) regulation 5 and schedules 1, 2 and 3 (Welsh Assembly Government 2007) sets out what the responsible authority must take into account when placing children outside the area where they live. The clinical nurse specialists for Looked After children are members of the panel of professionals who meet to make arrangements for the child placed outside the area, providing health advice and information.

There are efforts to bring children placed outside the borough back into the area where it is safe and appropriate to do so but this will take time. Children under the care of the Caerphilly social services department who are placed outside the Borough and outside the 20 mile perimeters covered by the nurses in Caerphilly access local services for their health assessments. This is coordinated for them by the health clerical support in Caerphilly overseen by the clinical nurse specialists. The children have their health assessment carried out by a medical officer or a nurse in the area where they live who sends the completed documents to the team in Caerphilly. The Caerphilly clinical nurse specialists then reviews the health assessment documents and ensures that the health action plan is completed before returning the forms to the child's social worker. We do this because of an audit which found that although health issues were documented on the health assessment forms from other areas they were not always highlighted in the health care plan. As it is the health care plan rather than the health assessment form which is available for the social services Looked After review, the children's health problems were often not appreciated by social workers, nor were there time scales or clarity about who was responsible for dealing with outstanding health issues.

The system of health and social services working together to undertake the initial Looked After health assessment
On reviewing health assessment arrangements for Looked After children in Caerphilly in the late 1990s it was clear that if the service was to become more child focused and

efficient there needed to be agreement between health and social services about professional responsibilities and the time scales to be adhered to. Our protocol is as follows.

- At the point of entry into the care system the child's social worker obtains parental consent for the Looked After health assessment to be carried out and for the exchange of information between health and social services.
- Social services has to get the 'proforma (document) of information' which includes the child's name, home and placement addresses, school, general practitioner and name of social worker to the health clerical support and the clinical nurse specialist within 48 hours of the child becoming Looked After.
- Social services have 72 hours to provide the health clerical support and the clinical nurse specialist with the consent. (The child has the right to ask for confidentiality and this is explained to them.)
- On receipt of the 'proforma of information' the health clerical support obtains the child's health records for the child. These include community records, paediatric records, school and health visiting records and child protection records.
- The health clerical support then makes an appointment for the child to have a Looked After health assessment within 2 weeks of the child becoming Looked After.
- The clinical nurse specialist reads the records and records the family and child's health history.
- The clinical nurse specialist sees the child and undertakes the health assessment at the placement address or at a health clinic near to where the child lives, 2 weeks after the child has become Looked After.
- At the health assessment various tools (see below) are used to gather health data. This involves looking at health from a holistic perspective.
- A health action plan is written, this includes details of which professional has responsibility for outstanding health and well-being issues and time scales for review. Referrals to other services or follow-up appointments before the next Looked After health assessment are highlighted.
- The health assessment form and the health action plan is sent to the social worker within 24 hours of the assessment being undertaken and therefore in time for the first social services Looked After review.
- The social worker takes the health action plan to the social services Looked After review where outstanding health issues are shared including who is responsible for addressing these.
- The recommendations from the social services review are sent to the clinical nurse specialists for Looked After children and the communication loop is complete.

The system for the Looked After health reviews
Once the child's details are entered into the health database the child is automatically recalled for the Looked After health assessment review. If the child returns home in the

interim social services inform the health clerical support of this with a second proforma and no health assessment review is arranged.

In Caerphilly health assessments are carried out at the following times:

1. For children under 5 years:
    - within 2 weeks of becoming Looked After, this fits into the National Service Framework standards for early intervention, and comprehensive assessment of a child and family (carer's) needs (DH 2004b);
    - 5 months later;
    - Every 6 months after this.

    This enables the health assessments to fit into social services Looked After reviews for the under 5 years.
2. For children over 5 years:
    - within 2 weeks of becoming Looked After;
    - 9 months later;
    - Thereafter annually.

    The child is seen as frequently as needed to address outstanding health issues.

Changes for social workers

The move away from the medical model of service for Looked After children to the nurse-delivered model was initially met with some concern from social workers. However, the new system has fostered a more integrated approach to health care. The clinical nurse specialists are more accessible to social workers than medical officers. We work (full time) with Looked After children and social workers can contact us directly regarding any Looked After child on their caseload. When a problem is found at the health assessment the social worker is contacted by phone, the issue discussed and agreement reached about who is responsible for ensuring that the child's needs are met. If health concerns arise between assessments the social worker knows we will see the child or contact the carer so that we can work together to meet the child's needs.

Our social service child care teams (we have seven different ones in our borough) report that communication between health and social services is better and the coordination of services has improved since the clinical nurse specialists service for Looked After children was introduced.

Over the years we have observed that foster carers and children welcome contact with us. Often we are the only constant professional in the child's care experience since Wales has difficulty in recruiting and retaining children's social workers. The Children's Commissioner for Wales report in 2004 commented that some children do not have an allocated social worker and that the high turnover of social workers meant some children having up to three social workers in a year (Children's Commissioner for Wales 2004).

The health assessment form
The health assessment form is a 10-page document that has been developed by the clinical team. The content of the form has evolved over the 8 years it has been in use. It is used for the initial and the review health assessment.

Once a child has been seen for a Looked After health assessment the information collected is entered into our database.

This information is then used for audit, monitoring, planning and developing services, and to inform social services of *Children First* targets (www.childrenfirst.wales. gov.uk). (The programme in England is *Quality Protects*, www.dcsf.gov.uk/quality protects.)

The health assessment form includes:

- the child details (name, date of birth, SSD (social services department) identifier and NHS numbers);
- as much information as possible of the family and the child's health history;
- the child's current state of health and development;
- place of birth, gestation, weight at birth, time of birth;
- past and current addresses, telephone contact details;
- name of school, attendance rate, extra help needed, problems at school;
- name, address and last contact with the general practitioner, dentist and optician;
- immunisation status and need for catch up where appropriate;
- ethnicity;
- care history date, when became Looked After, length of time in current placement;
- emotional well-being, using the Strengths and Differences Questionnaire (SDQ) and general questioning regarding the child's behaviour in placement, at school and socially;
- weight and height and for those under 1 year head circumference;
- the Schedule of Growing Skills (SOGS)(a developmental assessment for children under 5 years);
- functional and developmental assessment using SPOTRN (**S** satisfactory, **P** Problem, **O** Observed, **T** Treatment, **R** Referral, **N** not examined, from coding in the personal child health record);
- details of other professionals who were/are seeing or due to see the child;
- health damaging behaviours, e.g. smoking, alcohol and substance use;
- sexual health and contraception;
- contact with family members;
- health promotion, health education and health protection;
- siblings names, date of birth and addresses.

Tools used in health assessment

Assessment of emotional well-being and identifying mental health problems – the Strengths and Difficulties Questionnaire (SDQ) (Goodman and Scott 1999)
'Health is a basis for a good quality of life and mental health is of overriding importance in this' (Article 24 UN Convention, http://www.unhchr.ch/html/menu3/b/k2crc.htm). Recognition of emotional and behavioural problems in Looked After children and effective interventions is clearly of benefit to children and their foster carers and may also reduce the incidence of mental health problems in later life (Mental Health Foundation 1999).

Over recent times there have been concerns about the range of emotional, behavioural and mental health problems of children in the Looked After system. The risk of mental health problems is higher in Looked After children than in any other group of children (Bamford and Wolkind 1988) and studies have consistently shown that they have a high incidence of behavioural problems. McCann and colleagues (1996) found that Looked After adolescents are at a higher risk of psychiatric problems than those living in their own families. While some recover without specialist intervention, Smith (2002) reported that 'a worrying continuity has been observed between childhood problems and adult outcomes'. Clearly identifying emotional, behavioural and mental health problems in children entering the Looked After system should be a priority as should access to specialist help for those with difficulties. Worryingly, a study from the Maudsley Hospital (Phillips 1997) found that although social workers thought 80% of Looked After children had mental health problems only 27% were referred for therapy.

In the early 2000s we compared the ability of clinical nurse specialists to clinically identify mental health problems in children and young people being seen for a health assessment with the findings when the clinical nurse specialists used the Strengths and Difficulties Questionnaire (SDQ). Identification was better when the questionnaire was used. We now use the questionnaire as part of the initial health assessment for all Looked After children of comprehensive/secondary school age.

Assessing development – The Schedule of Growing Skills II (SOGS)
Children under the age of 5 years entering the Looked After system have an assessment of their development using the SOGS. This is either done by the clinical nurse specialist or the child's health visitor.

It identifies children with significant developmental delay who need to be discussed with the consultant paediatrician and be referred to other services (e.g. audiology) and for other children the assessment provides a baseline for monitoring developmental progress in the Looked After system.

The personal child health record (PCHR)
Every child who becomes Looked After is given a PCHR. The child/carer and/or family member is encouraged to use this between Looked After health assessments to record dental/vision, screening and other appointments for the child. Following each health

assessment a duplicate of the health action plan (which is also sent to social services) is entered into the PCHR.

Health promotion/health education/health protection
The identification and prevention of illness should be carried out alongside health screening and health promotion during Looked After health assessments (Hill and Watkins 2003).

Many studies have shown that children entering the Looked After system have had poor access to health services, poor uptake of child health surveillance and immunisation, little contact with the dental and ophthalmic services and received minimal health education.

The health problems of Looked After children are often rooted in their pre-care experiences and circumstances, many have come from families where:

- there are drug and alcohol problems;
- there is domestic violence;
- there are individuals with special needs, e.g. disability;
- the family functions poorly;
- the family has been mobile/had several address changes;
- there are mental health problems. (Howell 2001)

Often there are child protection concerns including abuse and neglect which may have been present for a number of years before the child entered the care system.

The role of the clinical nurse specialist is to be vigilant to the needs of this vulnerable group, to support other professionals and the foster carers in managing the children and disseminate information on 'a need to know' basis for the good of the child. It is helpful to remember the principles of the UN Convention on the Rights of the Child and the Welsh Assembly's Seven Core Aims for Children and Young People (http://www.allwales unit.gov.uk/media/pdf/d/s/cyp04-pt3-e.pdf). These are for children:

1   To have a flying start in life.
2   To have a comprehensive range of education and learning opportunities.
3   To enjoy the best possible health and be free from abuse, victimisation and exploitation.
4   To have access to play, leisure, sporting and cultural activities.
5   To be listened to, treated with respect, and have their race and cultural identity recognised.
6   To have a safe home and community that supports physical and emotional well-being.
7   Not to be disadvantaged by poverty.

We encourage children to take responsibility for their own health and to pursue a healthy lifestyle. If appropriate they may be encouraged to institute a small change by the time of their next health assessment e.g. to clean their teeth in the morning as well as the night or to try a small amount of a fruit or vegetable they think they won't like (some children have had minimal experience of fresh fruit and vegetables at home and imagine they will not like it). For older children a visit to a young people's sexual health clinic may be suggested or to try out activities at the leisure centre or to let us know how they get on reducing their cigarette smoking.

There is also a role for the clinical nurse specialists in educating Looked After children on personal health issues e.g. menstruation and sex education, particularly for those who may have missed out on this at school due to poor attendance or frequent changes of school. The clinical nurse specialists may need to liaise with the school nurse or teachers about such issues with the child's consent.

The role of the clinical nurse specialist in the multiagency team

Many of the problems facing Looked After disabled children are similar to those experienced by all children in the Looked After system. The disabled child often comes from a dysfunctional family where there has been a background of neglect and abuse.

Studies have shown that parents and carers of disabled children want a single point of contact for health issues (Gero et al 2004). The clinical nurse specialists is in a good position to act as the health 'coordinator' for the Looked After disabled child. Like others entering the Looked After system the health care of the disabled child may have become fragmented or the child may have become lost to medical follow-up.

There is a danger that disabled children are regarded as different from others in the Looked After system and that their impairment becomes their most prominent feature. We try as far as possible to treat them in the same way as other children while paying attention to their unique needs. In Caerphilly we use the same health assessment documents and processes for disabled children as for all Looked After children. They are given the same opportunities as other children regarding health protection and health promotion. Wherever possible the child contributes to the assessment and has their say in the care we are providing for them or in the services we contact on their behalf.

The Children Act (1989) puts a duty on local authorities to provide services to enable disabled children to lead as normal a life as possible. The UN Convention (Article 2.3) states that disabled children must be helped to be as independent as possible and be able to take a full and active part in everyday life. Through local knowledge and links with other health professionals involved with disabled children (therapists, dieticians, special school nurses, community paediatricians, neurologists), social services and education, the clinical nurse specialists is in a good position to ameliorate difficulties and to try and ensure the disabled child maximises their abilities and reaches their full potential (DH 2004c).

Training for foster carers

Over the years that we have been providing training for foster carers we have noticed changes in their perception of the clinical nurse specialists service for Looked After children. We have not audited this but anecdotal evidence suggests that foster carers were surprised at first when we didn't formally examine the child at the initial health assessment and when, in addition to asking about health matters, we also inquired about school, contact, feelings, social problems including involvement with the police, friendships, health damaging behaviours etc. Some foster carers felt many of these questions were inappropriate initially but all have changed their views after attending training sessions. We now find attendance for children's appointments is much improved, that foster carers are more involved with their children's leisure activities and that they encourage the children to take responsibility for their own health as far as is developmentally possible

Foster carers are now proactive in registering their foster child with a dentist, an optician and a general practitioner. Often they tell us at the initial health assessment (2 weeks after the child moved to their care) that the child is registered with a general practitioner and that they have dental and vision tests booked for the child!

We know many of the foster carers well. Our contact with them is not just limited to the children's health assessments and training sessions, we also respond to worries about their foster child whether this is a health, education or a social concern. We feel that anything that impacts upon the child's well-being needs addressing promptly; this may involve us contacting the children's rights officer or the education services or doing a piece of direct work with the carer, such as management of bedwetting. We believe it is important that foster carers are appreciated and supported in caring for children.

Chapter 5

Emotional and Developmental Issues for Disabled Children Who Live Away from Home

Annette Hames

Introduction

There is evidence that some disabled children are at increased risk of abuse, and that abuse itself further disables children and can lead to adverse emotional development. This chapter examines some of the reasons why disabled children are at risk, briefly summarizes how the infant brain develops and how impairments may be attributable to abuse and neglect, and describes the emotional effects that abuse and neglect can have on children. This is followed by a brief description of issues for children who are placed in residential settings because of their challenging needs, followed by a final section describing the best ways of managing disabled children who are living away from home.

Disability and abuse

Disabled children's vulnerability

Disabled children have particular issues that make them more vulnerable to abuse than other children. Three important issues are their:

- dependence on others;
- increased use of residential facilities; and
- communication needs.

Disabled children are often extremely dependent upon others for their personal care activities, such as bathing, dressing and toileting and these tasks may be delivered by a large number of others. Personal care may also have to continue for long periods of time, for some children throughout their childhood and into their adult years. Many disabled children use institutional care for short periods of respite, residential schooling, or long-term institutional care and there have been many documented incidents of abuse of disabled children in institutions. In the past there has been a tendency to deny that professionals who care for disabled children would abuse their position, and this in turn has made disabled children even more vulnerable. Finally, children's limited communication with others can make them especially vulnerable. Some of the most vulnerable children are those whose impairments prevent them from communicating. Disabled children may be unable to report abuse because they have received no sex education in special needs schools, may not have appropriate vocabularies if they use alternative forms of communication or feel shame or fear about reporting it. Child protection professionals are often unable to communicate with non-verbal children.

While there has been much investigation recently of the link between disability and abuse, there has also been criticism of many of these studies (Westcott and Jones 1999). This is because many include only small groups of children so it is unclear whether their findings would generalize to larger groups; studies have rarely used control groups to ensure that it is disability and not some other factor that is leading to abuse; and much of the research has been imprecise about how to define both disability and abuse. There appear to be conflicting reports about whether there is a relationship between the severity of disability and the risk of abuse, with some research suggesting that more disabled children are at greater risk of being abused, while others suggest that less disabled children are at greater risk (Westcott and Jones 1999). Recent reviews report that children with certain disabilities are at greater risk of abuse. Children with conduct disorder and learning disabilities appear to be at greatest risk. Children with cerebral palsy may be at increased risk of physical abuse and neglect, though the evidence for this link is fairly weak. Autism and sensory disorders do not seem to predispose to abuse (Govindshenoy and Spencer 2007).

While it is now clear that some disabled children are at high risk of being abused and will suffer emotionally as a result, a further confounding factor is that child abuse and disability are both linked with many other factors that place children at risk of developing psychological problems, including poverty, social isolation and general family stress (Westcott 1991). Therefore it must be recognized that the emotional responses of disabled children may not only occur as a result of abuse, but also be because of poverty, isolation or family stress, or from the experiences of being disabled in a society that discriminates against them (Kennedy 1990).

Normal brain growth
Many children are removed from home, during their early years, when their brain growth and development are at their most active. Brain development is constantly modified by the child's environment, and abuse and neglect are aspects that could adversely influence its development. Recently there has been increasing evidence for the neurobiological mechanisms by which abuse may be linked with behavioural and emotional impairment. While much of this work is still at a preliminary stage, evidence is accumulating for an association between exposure to childhood abuse and alterations in brain structure and functioning and possible psychopathology. There are some limitations to this research, as many studies have had small samples, some have had no control groups, many are animal studies, and those with children have

sometimes included children with multiple diagnoses and sometimes only children of one gender.

The volume of the human brain increases more during the first year of life than at any other time, from an average weight of 400 g to 1000 g at 12 months of age (Glaser, 2000). The brain contains many neurons (nerve cells) (See Figure 5.1) which communicate with each other by sending messages from the cell body (axon) of one neuron and receiving messages through the cell extension (dendrite) of another. The point where the axon and dendrite meet is called the synapse. Nerve impulses are carried across the synaptic gap by neurotransmitters. During the first 2 years of life, within the brain there is an overproduction of axons, dendrites and synapses, and subsequently many have to be 'pruned'. The most frequent and repetitive experiences and connections are reinforced, whereas those that are unused are pruned. In this way learning takes place and the brain takes shape.

The process by which the brain's structure and functions are altered in response to learning is referred to as 'neural plasticity'. Children's brains are particularly sensitive, take longer to mature compared with other animals, and during this period can be particularly vulnerable to unusual environmental experiences. There is increasing neurological evidence to show that various stressful events, such as child abuse, provoke stress responses in the brain that result in abnormalities in the pruning process and subsequently lead to adverse emotional reactions.

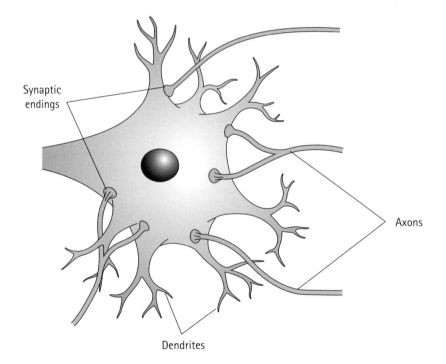

Synaptic endings

Axons

Figure 5.1
A neuron

Dendrites

Hormonal changes occur in the brain as a response to stress. Cells in an area of the brain known as the hypothalamus secrete chemicals known as neuropeptides to another area of the brain called the pituitary gland. They stimulate further chemicals called adrenocorticotropic hormone (ACTH). This chemical is carried through the bloodstream to the adrenal glands, where they trigger production and release of the stress hormone called cortisol. This whole system is called the HPA-axis (hypothalamus–pituitary–adrenal cortex) (see Figure 5.2). In another area of the brain, called the brain stem, lies the sympathetic nervous system which stimulates the release of adrenaline as part of the 'fight/flight' response. Both chemicals, cortisol and adrenaline, generate extra energy and mobilize the body for action. The parasympathetic nervous system reduces reactivity to threats. The HPA-axis has to be regulated so that it is only activated when needed then returns to normal levels. Frequent stress activation, with prolonged cortisol production, can result in impaired brain growth and organization, and can also chronically suppress immune functioning, increasing the child's vulnerability to infectious diseases. Both low and high levels of brain reactivity are associated with poor mental and emotional health, whereas moderate reactivity is associated with adaptive functioning.

Environmental influences on brain growth
It has been suggested that in a stress-filled world, children form alternative neurological pathways as adaptations to high levels of stress hormones. This then allows maltreated children to protect themselves, by developing an acutely sensitive fight/flight response system. However, a change that has been adaptive in the context of a high-stress

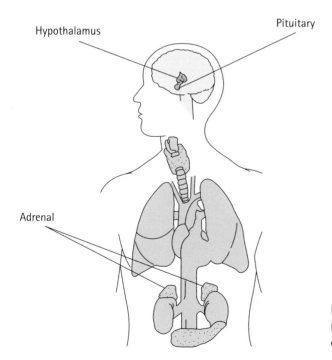

Hypothalamus

Pituitary

Adrenal

Figure 5.2 The HPA–axis (hypothalamus–pituitary–adrenal cortex)

environment becomes maladaptive in the normal environment, and increases the risk of serious health problems and psychopathology (Gunnar 2007).

The hippocampus, amygdala and corpus callosum are areas of the brain that have a long period of postnatal development and are therefore particularly vulnerable to the effects of stress and early maltreatment (Ayoub and Rappolt-Schlichtmann 2007). The hippocampus is involved in verbal memory. It has a long postnatal developmental period, and high density of cortisol receptors. There is some evidence that children who have been abused have a reduction in left hippocampal volume which is associated with encoding and retrieving memory difficulties and problems with inhibition of distracting information. Children who have been abused may present with poor memory, be distractible and experience intrusive painful memories.

The amygdala is involved in emotions, and particularly fear and vigilance. There has been some suggestion that there is a reduction in amygdala volume and abnormal amygdala activity among children who have been abused. As the amygdala consolidates the emotional significance of traumatic events, altered functioning may result in increased negativity, dissociation and hypervigilance or numbing of affect as abused children are unable to manage painful emotions.

The corpus callosum connects both hemispheres of the brain, the left hemisphere (which is dominant for logical abilities) with the right hemisphere (which is dominant for spatial and visual abilities). The corpus callosum is responsible for integrating communication between both hemispheres. It has been found to be reduced in size in some abused children, thereby diminishing the communication between the cortical hemispheres. It has been suggested that children who have been abused have difficulty integrating information and split their memories, particularly when these have emotional content. They have difficulties merging positive and negative memories, with a strong bias towards their negative memories. They also find it difficult to integrate information when problem solving (Ayoub and Rappolt-Schlichtmann 2007, Teicher et al 2006).

Attachment

Attachment is vital to child development and is affected by abuse and neglect. There is also evidence that a child's attachment status will influence their developing neurological response to stress.

Attachment refers to the relationship between the child and his or her primary caregiver and forms the basis for a child's long-term positive relationships with others. A child needs an attachment with an adult who is both nurturing and protective, and who fosters trust and security. Attachment was first described by Bowlby (1969) as a biological instinct. As the infant becomes closer to his or her attachment figure, whether this is a parent or the primary carer, this attachment figure is able to reduce any form of stress. The response of the primary caregiver to the child's attachment needs helps the child to construct internal models of themselves and their carer. These models then become the beliefs that the child holds about him or herself and form predictions about how he or she will be treated in the future by others.

Attachment status is measured, usually during a child's first year, using a well-validated measure called the strange situation procedure (Ainsworth et al 1978). Using this measure, four categories of attachment have been observed and defined, one described as secure and three as insecure.

1. Securely attached infants (B) have internal models of caregivers as consistent and supportive, show distress when the caregiver leaves, and can be comforted when this person returns.
2. Anxious/avoidant insecurely attached infants (A) try to protect themselves by showing little overt indications of emotional distress when left.
3. Anxious/resistant insecurely attached infants (C) become extremely distressed when the caregiver leaves and are difficult to settle when this person returns.
4. Disorganized/disoriented insecurely attached infants (D) have no strategies for dealing with their distress and will both approach and avoid others in order to try and deal with their distress.

Generally, more sensitive parents have more securely attached children. This is the case with children with learning disabilities and language delays, though less so in children with autism, who tend to show more disorganized attachments, even with sensitive parenting. There is also an over-representation of disorganized attachments among children with learning disabilities (van Ijzendoorn et al 2007).

It has been found that over 80% of abused 12-month old infants fall into the disorganized category compared with approximately 20% of non-abused infants (Carlson et al 1989). It is suggested that this is because abused children are unable to feel secure, but instead become frightened, disorganized and disorientated as they seek comfort from their primary attachment figures, who at the same time are their abusers.

Most studies of insecure attachment status have been carried out with children who have been physically abused and/or neglected, and not with children who have been sexually abused. It may be that neglect, emotional abuse and physical abuse are most likely to be perpetrated by the child's primary caregiver, thereby affecting their attachment status, whereas it is likely that sexual abuse will be perpetrated by someone who is not the primary carer (Glaser 2000). Therefore it may be that children who have been sexually abused can still be securely attached.

Effects of child abuse and neglect
A number of longitudinal studies, following the progress of children over time, have shown a strong association between abuse and neglect and subsequent social, emotional, behavioural and cognitive impairments.

The Minnesota Mother–Child Project (Erickson and Egeland 1996) is a longitudinal study that has followed a large group of children born to first time mothers who have been identified as at-risk for parenting problems. Abused and neglected children showed developmental delay and delayed expressive and receptive language, social interaction problems, poor coping strategies and difficulties with emotion regulation. Interestingly, neglect occurring in the absence of other forms of abuse, resulted in worse outcomes for children than neglect occurring alongside physical abuse. Other studies have also found that neglect alone is more detrimental to expressive and receptive language than physical abuse or abuse and neglect together (Allen and Oliver 1982). It may be that physical contact in the form of abuse is less harmful than neglect and no contact at all, when parents are more emotionally detached and less interested in their children. During their school-age years, neglected children presented with more internalizing problems (such as depression and anxiety) while physically abused children presented with more externalizing problems (such as behavioural problems).

The Bucharest Early Intervention Project (Nelson et al 2007) was an opportunity to observe the restorative effects of foster care on later development. Many children were institutionalized in Romania when this project started and foster care did not exist. The authors developed their own system of foster care, and a group of institutionalized children were randomly assigned to be placed in foster care while others remained in institutions. The children were aged between 5 and 31 months at the start of the study and were followed through to the age of 54 months.

- It was found that physical, cognitive, linguistic and socioemotional development were all severely affected by institutional rearing.
- There was a substantial increase in emotional and behavioural difficulties among the institutionalized group (50%) whereas a never-institutionalized group (in Romania) presented with disorders that were similar to populations in North America.
- The institutionalized children also showed more disorganized attachments, being more emotionally withdrawn and socially disinhibited.

Following placement, the children in foster care made significant cognitive gains over the institutionalized group, but were not able to reach the level of the never-institutionalized group. Foster care reduced the frequency of depression and anxiety though did not appear to have any effect on externalizing symptoms such as attention-deficit–hyperactivity disorder (ADHD) and disruptive behaviour. While the foster care group no longer showed signs of emotional withdrawal, they were still socially disinhibited. The findings support the notion of sensitive periods for early brain development, and if placement in foster care occurs too late, the child will not be able to recover. While there may be some recovery in cognitive abilities, impairments in attachment, behaviour and language may be harder to improve if children have been in neglectful or abusive settings for too long.

Other studies looking at UK adoptions from Romanian orphanages have also found adopted children to be seriously delayed in their cognitive and social functioning. Their cognitive progress following adoption was predicted by the age when they were adopted, with adoption before 6 months of age appearing to be protective of later developmental delay (Rutter et al 1998).

There is some evidence of adult repercussions for children who have a history of physical and sexual abuse. For example, there is a higher incidence of post-traumatic stress disorder (PTSD) in Vietnam veterans who have experienced childhood physical abuse (Bremner et al 1993).

The importance of secure and positive attachments
It has been suggested that one function of the secure attachment relationship is to protect the developing brain from the potential negative effects of increased cortisol on the brain during stressful moments and particularly during the vulnerable first 2 years of postnatal brain development (Gunnar 2007).

- Babies tend to have low levels of cortisol for the first few months, as long as sensitive carers help them maintain their equilibrium through touch, feeding and rocking, but their immature systems are unstable and can easily be overwhelmed. Psychosocial stressors, such as brief separations from the caregiver and childhood inoculations, have been found to produce elevations in cortisol levels before, but not after 1 year of age.
- One-year-olds with insecure attachments show raised cortisol levels when first attending childcare with their mothers, compared with secure toddlers. Once mothers leave, the cortisol levels of both securely and insecurely attached toddlers become similarly raised, indicating that they are both stressed. Even mild everyday stressors (such as being picked out of the bath) have been shown to produce elevations in cortisol levels that are more quickly reduced by sensitive maternal caring (Albers et al 2008).

A secure attachment relationship during infancy can therefore protect the developing brain from the potential negative affects of prolonged increased cortisol levels.

It has been suggested that positive attachments may help restore some of the neurobiological alterations that have occurred as a result of early abuse (Gunnar 2007; Rick and Douglas 2007). Many children who have been removed from home because of abuse, later have a history of multiple placements. The availability of a supportive or alternative carer has been demonstrated to be one of the most important factors that distinguish abused children with good developmental outcomes from those who have poorer outcomes. Gunnar has pointed out that there is great plasticity in children's brains that allows for the potential for adaptation in the brain towards more normative states and patterns following transition to more responsive care.

Children who live away from home for other reasons
It has been estimated that at least 12% of children with disabilities are likely to be looked after away from home for 90 days or more each year (McConkey et al 2004). Attendance at residential school is the most common reason for living away from home, at the same time that there has been a general decline in placing children without disabilities into residential care. In McConkey's sample:

- 51% of children had severe learning disabilities;
- 29% had profound learning or multiple disabilities;
- 10% had mild or moderate learning disabilities; and
- 10% had physical disabilities.
- 14% of the children were classed as technologically dependent, including children who required tube feeding, regular blood transfusions or ventilation
- nearly half had challenging behaviour;
- a third had severe communication problems;
- nearly one-fifth had autism spectrum disorders.

Parents' experiences prior to placing their children in residential schooling have universally been reported as negative and stressful (McGill et al 2006). They have described feeling isolated and excluded from professional advice and services. As their children's needs increase, so they have been excluded from precisely those services that are supposed to provide support, including respite and local schooling. Related to these difficulties, parents have frequently reported that their children have been neglected. Traumatic family experiences are certain to have interfered with children's emotional development and exacerbated any challenging behaviours. However, there has been very limited investigation of the emotional experiences of disabled children living in residential care. Some children have reported feeling homesick while others have described how residential school allows them to make friends and be more independent (Abbott et al 2001). However, views have not been gathered from the majority of disabled children who are placed in residential schooling and who have limited abilities to express themselves as a result of their communication problems or profound disabilities.

Sensitive care for disabled children who live away from home
There is increasing evidence that, due to the neural plasticity of young children's brains and the potential for brain structures to adapt as a result of environmental changes, children's behaviour and emotional reactions can change as a result of moves to more sensitive and responsive care. The earlier this occurs and the less abusive the child's experiences have been, the more likely it is that the child is able to make a successful adaptation.

If carers are well informed about the child's past experiences and the likely effects that these could have upon emotional and behavioural progress, then they may be more tolerant of slow progress and setbacks to progress. It will also help carers if they have accurate knowledge of the child's disability and likely prognosis. Child care professionals do not always have this information and it may be necessary to gain advice from professionals in the disability field. Carers will benefit from knowing the importance of the environment on the development of normal brain functioning. Children are generally helped by being provided with nurturance and love, stability and predictability.

While some carers may believe or hope that they can make a difference to a child, just by placing him or her in an alternative and more positive and secure environment, there needs to be recognition that disabled children who have been abused still need the same clear management and guidelines as other disabled children. Carers of disabled children, both natural parents and foster parents, often state that they 'feel sorry' for children with disabilities, make allowances for them, not treating them with the same clear guidance and support that they provide for their other children. Children with disabilities, particularly if they have cognitive delays, have difficulties picking up the subtle cues of how to behave, and therefore need tighter guidance rather than carers being more lax. Lack of clarity can confuse children.

If the disabled child has any degree of cognitive or language delay, one of the most important aspects of managing and dealing with his or her emotions and behaviour involves being able to understand the child's developmental level. While a child may be at a certain chronological level, carers must recognize that language needs to be directed towards the child at a level that he or she can understand. It is therefore important that professionals involved with the child assess the child's cognitive and linguistic level and pass this information on to direct carers. If this information is not available, carers may interpret any unresponsiveness or misbehaviour on the part of the child as due to disobedience when it is actually due to lack of comprehension. For example, a child who has a chronological age of 5 years but a comprehension level of 2 years, will not understand complex instructions and demands. Instructions will need to be given in clear, brief and precise ways; only one or two words may be needed. The child may be confused by negative commands, and find it easier to understand when they are told what to do rather than what not to do.

Whether or not children have visual or auditory impairments, they are likely to have attentional difficulties, particularly if they are developmentally delayed. Therefore communication must be directed to them from close by, sometimes even at the child's physical level, with clear eye contact and by using the child's name. Other distractions should be reduced, for example televisions turned off and other children removed from the area when having to concentrate. Carers need to be aware that at times of emotional intensity, for example when children are angry or upset, their comprehension level will decrease, and therefore carers will need to be more clear, brief and precise. A long tirade from the carer will not be understood by an emotionally upset and developmentally delayed child.

It is vital that carers are consistent. This means not only that behaviour management and guidelines from one carer are applied consistently, but there is consistency across carers. This is particularly important for children who are cared for by multiple carers and for children who have been abused and have insecure attachments. Consistency makes boundaries clearer, and provides security for children who are developmentally delayed and who have come from disorganized environments. Abused and developmentally delayed children with disorganized attachments will test boundaries to the full.

Carers may need professional support to recognize the impact of a child's previous experiences and relationships upon current relationships, and the intense feelings that may be projected to or from the child. A child's previous attachment history will affect their current interactions.

- Children with disorganized attachments will need carers who are clear in their boundaries and who can tolerate the child's variability and unpredictability.
- An avoidant child will be very slow in forming relationships, always anticipating rejection.
- Children who have been physically abused may expect aggression and may work towards provoking it. This can be extremely frustrating for carers, who may end up feeling that the child is deliberately manipulating them.
- A child who has been sexually abused is likely to continue to behave in a sexually inappropriate way with other members of the family, despite constant reminders that this is not appropriate behaviour.
- Developmentally delayed children may show sexualized behaviours that are well beyond their developmental level. These behaviours can be especially draining for carers and can cause further problems, particularly if children are in settings with other disabled children.

This is where it is important that professionals who are experienced in working with abused children and those who work with disabled children need to work together to support carers. When children have been severely abused at a very early developmental stage, carers need to fully understand where the behaviour has come from. If carers are supported to understand the basis of behaviours then they are more likely to be sympathetic towards the child, and less likely to project their anger onto him or her.

Finally, it may be appropriate that some disabled children who have been abused are referred on for professional help. Child psychotherapy will be appropriate for some children. Some will benefit from behavioural strategies to help them gain control over their environment. Cognitive methods for building self-esteem have also been found to be effective in helping abused children adapt positively to their environment.

Box 5.1 Case study

Julie was a severely intellectually disabled 7-year-old, who had been sexually abused by her mother before the age of 2, placed in foster care at 3, and then further sexually abused by her foster carer. She was now living with her second foster carer and attending a school for children with severe and profound learning difficulties. Her intellectual abilities were at the level of a 5-year-old, though in addition, she had severe expressive language difficulties that made her very difficult to understand. She required constant supervision, could not be left to go to the toilet on her own, and needed close supervision when changing for physical education lessons as she would try and touch the other children. She was making very slow progress with her language and social skills, and was very self-conscious of her limited expressive skills.

A child psychotherapist who had previously assessed Julie, worked with her carer and school staff and explained some of Julie's background to them. Staff had been unaware of the details of her early abuse, and were then able to understand where her sexualized behaviours had come from. They also gained some understanding of the disorganization of her early years and how this impacted on her later unpredictability. It became clear that her early attachments had been very disorganized and that she constantly needed very clear boundaries and guidelines in order to help her feel safe. School staff recognized that Julie needed to re-experience her early years again, in a safe setting, and so offered her frequent opportunities to play with the early years toys that were available in the classroom for the more profoundly disabled children. Whenever Julie was expected to use language, she was offered the opportunity to use visual aids as well, to lessen the likelihood that she would feel self-conscious about her limited expressive skills.

Chapter 6

Management of Emotional and Behavioural Problems

Tom Berney

Introduction

The process of placement away from home will select children and adolescents who have psychological difficulties. These will be as varied as the children chosen, yet there are some common threads. It may be the child's disability making it difficult for the parents to provide 'good enough' care; difficulties in the parental personalities and relationships; or an interactive combination of both that leads to a child's move away from home. Removed from parents and family, the child is being cared for by professional substitutes that should bring the advantages of parenting by carers who are detached and have expertise, confidence and freshness but the arrangement may be undermined by economy and inexperience. Furthermore, whether the placement is in a hospital, residential school or foster home, the professionals are working within institutions, ranging from the partial to the total (examples of the latter being an institution for young offenders or the unit for a child whose fragile autism requires round-the-clock, consistent and structured care) that are subject to the hazards and strengths of institutions (Goffman 1990). These develop their own culture, often religiously employing a theoretical framework derived solely from a behavioural or a psychodynamic philosophy, that is used to understand the world and, within it, the child's behaviour, feelings and relationships.

What leads to the placement?

For some the move is to a centre that can provide for their educational needs often with the focus on a particular disability such as autism, epilepsy, cerebral palsy, communication difficulties or learning disabilities. For others the move is to resolve disturbance or to salvage some situation where the child or their environ is at risk. Here, in theory, the placement brings a more measured, professional approach compared with a home where parents, handicapped by the limitations of their accommodation, their neighbours and their surrounds, enmeshed in family ties, tired by the unbroken responsibility and hampered by the demands of other children, struggle to be consistent, fair and dispassionate. It would seem easy to improve on such a mix of disadvantage and much can be remedied by an effective home intervention programme. However, for some, disturbance may be so intense or entrenched or else relationships so irredeemably exhausted as to need the child to be looked after away from home.

The advent of inclusion and better local resources have reduced the demand for the more straightforward educational placement so that residential schools and colleges are being referred an increasingly disturbed population. The effect has been to shift the emphasis from the academic to the pastoral with programmes of intensive and consistent treatment, containing and managing a degree of disturbance that may be so extreme as to be a danger to the staff, peers or to the child itself.

Prevention

Disturbance can be minimized or even prevented by a thoughtful and objective approach to the care of the child. This entails a systematic review of the elements that make up the child's world from which should follow a formal plan for the child's care.

The elements that make up the system of care are:

1. The child – although the child's disabilities and disturbance may dominate discussion, a central issue must be how the child is going to maintain and develop stable, long-term relationships.
2. The family – what is the nature of their relationships with the child, both now and in the future. A recurrent hazard is an unintended, unilateral and unspoken detachment by the family (Baker et al 1993) that leaves the child guessing as to where they stand.
3. The carers – their personalities, confidence, training and level of skill. Within any placement, limited by shifts and leave rotas as well as by staff turnover, there should be one or two people available to the child, clearly identified and whose work allows room for a relationship to develop and be protected.
4. The framework of care – a well-managed system of care will ensure sufficient support and training for the staff to feel confident as well as to be competent. Supervision has to be sufficient to prevent abuse or a slow drift into unwitting idiosyncrasy – whether on a campus or in the community, an institution can slip readily into an isolated culture only for this to become starkly apparent in the relief of a newspaper exposé. For example, withdrawal from pleasurable activities (timeout) can easily turn into segregation (the child being kept apart from others) and seclusion (the child being kept on their own within a room against their will), particularly if the process is encouraged by a child who, for whatever reason, prefers to avoid their peers. It is easy to underestimate what is being asked of the system of care when it has to cope with unusual and extreme forms of behaviour. For example, violence (notably biting) can make staff wary of any contact, and self-injury (such as eye gouging or headbanging carried through to the extent that they threaten blindness) can elicit unusual and controversial responses. If a system is to

retain a normal perspective there has to be regular, open contact with people who are outside it. Lay people, such as visiting managers or school governors, are essential but, faced with unusual behaviour, these often lack the expertise and confidence to challenge a fluent carer. It is essential therefore that there is also input from independent professionals and, whether they are the child's social worker, psychologist or paediatrician, their contact has to be frequent enough and detailed enough for them to understand the care the child is receiving and to make useful comment: a half-yearly review does not give sufficient access to the child's world. It is also essential that there is a forum for discussion of any method that seems unusual – 'unusual' being measured best by what you would think were you to read of it being used somewhere else. Finally, if they are to be accountable, those with overall administrative responsibility, whether the directors of a company, trustees of a charity, or members of a local authority committee, must be aware of the techniques being used, not as abstract generalization but in concrete detail. Two traits can hinder carers. The first is a theoretical framework that is applied to all situations. It is rare that 'one size fits all' and people often need to be encouraged to consider what other reasons there might be for a child's behaviour. The second is the use of technical formulations, unleavened by everyday explanation; for example, while attachment theory may well explain a child's distress, 'homesickness' may be of more use to the person who is working with the child.

5.   Peer relationships – the part played by these in amplifying or improving a child's disturbance is so complex as to encourage people to overlook its importance. Bullying, often so subtle as to be unnoticed, needs active measures such as a buddy system, very close adult supervision and other specifics to control it (Besag 1989).

Whatever the circumstances leading to a move there should be a care plan that, to avoid convenient ambiguity, must be written and then regularly revised once the child is in the placement. The format will vary with the service but it should cover the following areas:

1.   An account of the child that includes, besides a general description of the child's circumstances and characteristics, information about their abilities. Here is the chance to forestall the assumptions that can exacerbate or even cause disturbance; for example, an overestimate of ability that leaves a child with a sense of failure and resentment as they struggle to cope or an underestimate that results in boredom and disruptive behaviour. The distinction between cognitive potential (as measured by IQ tests) and functional ability (quantified by scales such as the Vineland (de Bildt et al 2005)) is not always appreciated nor is the degree of difficulty that can arise from specific developmental disabilities, particularly in language. This last can be so misleading that it is worth setting out, systematically and in writing, a summary of the child's capacity for both comprehension and expression, in all modalities, verbal and non-verbal.

This description of the child is often set out in simple terms as a 'passport' that the child can use to introduce themselves to strangers.

2.　Why the child is moving:

    a.　the background to the move in sufficient detail to allow the new carers to understand the child's perspective when things unexpectedly start to go wrong;

    b.　the child's mental and physical health and their presentation, including:

- a diagnostic formulation,
- the degree of risk that this brings – to the child and to those around,
- their medication;

    c.　the aims of this placement:

- what should the placement achieve – in what ways do the views of the child, the family and the various professionals differ?
- the key personnel – both administrative and those responsible for day to day care. Who should the parents liaise with and how (e.g. if by telephone then how often and at what times)?
- the programmes of management/treatment that are to be used and for how long – what are the outcome targets – what personnel will these involve?
- what precautions need to be taken? Examples are the supervision of a child who may set fires, abscond or who sexualizes social relationships; chaperonage for staff working with a child who might make unfounded accusations of abuse; or building alterations for someone who is unusually destructive;

    d.　the duration of this placement – whether this is a short-term transition or a longer placement that will allow the development of stable relationships;

    e.　ideas about, and plans for, subsequent placement. Uncertainty about when and where a child is going next undermines any placement as well as prolonging it;

    f.　contingencies for predictable crises.

3.　Who is involved in the child's care:

    a.　the addresses and telephone numbers of all the professionals and family members that are involved with the child;

    b.　arrangements for continued contact with the child's family. The plan should stipulate when and how contact will occur as well as with whom. The degree of detail will depend on the circumstances but, if necessary, might set out how frequently there should be contact by telephone, who initiates the calls and when. The state of existing relationships must be checked regularly and actively managed where necessary, for example, by coaching and supporting parents, structuring their contact and arranging additional home visits. Contact must be tailored to the child's needs rather than governed by a system's routine or tradition.

4.　The legal basis for the child's care:

    a.　who is responsible for what decisions (e.g. to give psychotropic medication, to be referred to a psychiatrist or to have an operation) – how far does responsibility remain with the parents and what happens in the event of a dispute between them?

b. what is the child's ability to give and withhold consent for various levels of decision?

c. is the child subject to any constraint under legislation such as the Children Act, the Criminal Justice Act or the Mental Health Act; for example, is the child subject to a Guardianship or a Probation Order?

5. Where and when the child is moving into the placement:

a. with whom are they travelling and how?

b. what preparation should the child have for the placement and what will happen in reality. While the ideal is that the child should arrive well prepared and looking forward to the placement, in practice circumstances and prejudice frequently prevent this. Emergency is the most valid reason for an abrupt, unexpected move; convenience or incompetence (whether in the staff or the system) the most frequent. The approach needs to be flexible and tailored to the individual. For example, the usual preparation for a move may be intolerable for someone whose autism makes it difficult to appreciate a time frame. For them it might be better to have a series of preliminary social visits to become familiar with the building, staff and peers without knowing that it is intended that they might eventually stay there.

6. The views of the child and their family:

a. particularly important are those areas in which their views differ from those of the professional staff as well as those in which they differ from each other. There must be constant feedback and checks to make sure that someone who is overawed, inarticulate or angry is not ignored;

b. does the child have an advocate[1]; should there be an advocate; and are there any plans to obtain the services of an advocate?

The preparation of a care plan is a substantial exercise and much of the detail may seem unreasonably bureaucratic but shortcomings often become apparent only when disturbance develops.

Assessment

Disturbed behaviour covers the gamut of child and adolescent psychiatry and can be the outward sign of a number of underlying factors ranging from developmental disorders to emotional disorder or psychosis. Limited or distorted communication encourages

---

1 An advocate, in this context, is someone who is not necessarily legally qualified but simply a person who is independent and whose role is to put the child's view and wishes. This may range from merely interpreting what the child is saying through to deducing what, on the basis of their knowledge of the child, the child would have said if they were able to express a view. The advocate needs to know the child well and to have no personal interest in the decision.

much to be inferred about subjective experience making it difficult to disentangle the innate from environmental response. The combination of limited evidence with a convincing theoretical framework encourages diagnostic formulation on a par with fortune-telling.

Any episode of disturbance must be viewed in the context of the past history; sometimes suppressed in a wish to give a child a fresh start or to avoid a self-fulfilling label. It may be the continuance of a well-established pattern, a natural shift in someone with a cyclical career of good and bad spells, or the end of a lull created by the novelty of the placement (the 'honeymoon' phenomenon). Alternatively, the episode may represent an anxiety state, even amounting to panic or psychosis, in a child who has been destabilized by a move that entailed separation from familiar, attachment figures, a (relatively) secure base or an established routine. The degree of distress will be greater if the child has cause to worry about what is happening at home and this may be heightened by uncertainty for it is usually better to know the worst than to think about what might be happening.

Physical disorder must be excluded; ailments such as hay fever, toothache or earache, intercurrent infection or epilepsy may cause discomfort and thereby disturbance. Medication, particularly the psychotropic and antiepileptic drugs, can cause unexpected and idiosyncratic responses particularly in this population. Even where a prescription is well established, the change of placement can bring a change of formulation or of compliance so that the child may be taking the full dose of the drug for the first time.

The relationship between the child and the staff is one of the most difficult elements to assess. An analysis of incidents – when, in what circumstances and with whom they occur – can throw light on positive as well as negative relationships. While the system will describe staffing patterns in terms of resources, expertise and staff needs (e.g. 'he can cope with violence'), it is important to go past this to see things from the child's point of view. For example, consistency, familiarity, confidence and warmth can combine to make the child feel that they are wanted in a non-intrusive, safe and predictable relationship while the converse can produce disturbance.

Treatment

Choice of placement
This is complicated. Social stigma or family guilt may lead parents to oppose or undermine substitute parenting while accepting a residential school, ostensibly for specialist education. However, schools have holidays (although some provide placements for 50, or even 52, weeks a year) so that another base is still required. Behaviour that is very dangerous (such as fire-setting) may preclude school placement. Violent, destructive or sexualized behaviour may be difficult for a foster placement to cope with, particularly where there are other, vulnerable children in the home. However, rather than magnifying such problems, the child's disabilities can override them, providing a passport to specialist placements and funding.

The level or duration of disturbance may merit admission to a psychiatric inpatient unit. Statutory and insurance limitations make it difficult for anywhere else to cope with behaviour such as fire-setting, extreme self-injury, sexual offending and severe or persistent violence, particularly where medication or intensive individual therapy are part of the therapeutic response. In addition, the unit can provide the highest levels of structure and consistency in care as well as allowing the use of a legal framework to hold the child where parental ambivalence or their child's competence makes detention difficult (Berney 2000). Functioning well, the inpatient unit can improve children to the point where, even if a return to their own homes is not practicable, other out-of-home placements become possible. All the same, such placements are scarce and expensive so that there is the risk that the psychiatric unit turns into a safe place to store children while the community service deals with other, more immediate priorities. An agreed exit route is an essential part of the pre-admission care plan as, with its ever changing population of numerous staff and disturbed peers, the psychiatric unit is a long way from being the domestic setting that a child should have as a secure base, even as a temporary measure.

It can be difficult to find a suitable psychiatric unit. Few mainstream units are comfortable with disabilities that bring unusual modes of communication, forms of disorder in which their experience (and therefore expertise) is limited, and a child who may be vulnerable in the context of their usual patient population. For example, an adolescent unit in which the programme is based on peer group relationships, verbal therapies and abstract concepts may be harmful to someone with a learning disability or autism.

An alternative approach is to extend the role of the specialist school with dedicated input from other agencies to develop its expertise, staffing and physical surround. However, by taking on increasing levels of disturbance, the school risks becoming less suitable for the non-disturbed child who simply requires specialist education.

The child begins to develop multiple bases – divisions between care and education can exist in a residential school as well as between (foster) home and school. Holidays, even when limited to the Christmas/New Year fortnight, can be profoundly disruptive for a child who has little ability to cope with change or uncertainty and, consequently, whose greatest need is consistency.

Parents, relieved of the immediate worry of caring for their children, can become very prescriptive as to what treatments should be used or what they will allow, tying the hands of the staff to the point that the placement may become unsustainable. Work with parents is so essential that, while many rely on the statutory agencies, some placements employ their own social worker whose approach may range from family-centred casework to conjoint family therapy. This work, pre-dating any decision to move the child, will change its focus as the child moves into and through the placement and will need to deal with subsequent transitions. The parents might need help to cope with their guilt from allowing their child to move away from home (Baker and Blacher 2002; Green 2004) as well as their resentment at the stigma that this carries and their doubts about the ability of anyone else to care effectively for the child.

Use of medication

The use of psychotropic medication is always controversial although its merits in epilepsy and attention-deficit–hyperactivity disorder (ADHD) are accepted. Outside these (apparently) clear cut indications, doubts arise because of the child's developmental immaturity, inability to give consent and the potential for long-term use if the drug is effective. The limited market for drug sales means that there is little commercial point in applying for a prescribing licence so that, in this field, most drugs are used outside the manufacturer's licence. There are few randomized controlled trials, the evidential base largely consisting of a series of open-label trials that are often discarded in the preparation of guidelines that simply resort to advising against the use of the drug. All this makes it daunting to use medication until the cost (in terms of potential adverse effects) is clearly outweighed by the benefits. To take a common example: as with all drugs, wider use has led to the recognition that the newer, atypical neuroleptics have more adverse effects than previously thought; yet they can sometimes transform an irritable and unhappy child with autism, in constant confrontation with the world, into someone who is happier and able to enjoy their life. On the other hand, the result may be a fat, sleepy and dystonic child. The equation becomes more complicated when this makes the difference between a child staying in a domestic placement and a move to containment in a specialist hospital unit.

What drugs are helpful and when (Santosh and Baird 1999)? Outside the psychoses, psychiatric prescribing tends to target symptoms rather than disorders and, particularly in this population, where idiosyncratic responses are the rule, every prescription becomes a therapeutic trial. This is acceptable provided this is clear to everyone involved; the dosage starts at the lowest level practical and increases slowly ('start low, go slow') and there is a readiness to withdraw the drug if it is ineffective or uncomfortable. The restlessness and anxious arousal that indicate a drug-induced akathisia are commonly missed. The loss of confidence in therapist and drug that follows dyskinesia can justify the routine use of an anticholinergic drug (such as orphenadrine) to prevent its occurrence.

Ethical issues

Dealing with violence

Violence brings its own problems (Harris et al 1996; Department for Education and Skills and the Department of Health 2002), not simply as to its practical management but also in the legitimacy of the methods employed (Lyon and Pimor 2004). How far can a placement go in making demands and insisting that the child engage in everyday life? If someone is violently distressed, injuring either themselves or others, how far should they be allowed to become isolated; at what point should a hermit be allowed to adopt his/her vocation? While all staff should be taught how to avoid and to reduce aggression, should they be taught systematic physical responses, 'control and restraint' techniques? The intention is to give sufficient confidence to raise the threshold at which they resort to a physical response; learning the technique being akin to the lion-tamer's purchase of a pistol. However, it carries the risk of encouraging the staff to respond to violence with trained violence. While the use of injected medication belongs to the hospital setting, oral medication (such as chlorpromazine) can be authorised by a doctor by telephone and, given as syrup, can be nearly as rapid in its effect, the speed of absorption being increased by the addition of sugar (many syrups being sugar-free). Buccal neuroleptics are surer but, if swallowed, no faster than other oral preparations.

Programmes that use punishers, whether black marks or more physically aversive responses such as lemon sprays, electric shocks or loud noise (a shouted 'no'), can be very effective. The consequences, both for the child and for the staff, are so complex that they are best avoided although it remains open to debate whether they are warranted for extreme behaviour that is causing serious physical harm after all other measures have failed (Jacobson 1993). At an everyday level, the boundary becomes blurred between this and a reward-based programme. Depending on the child's response, it can be difficult to prevent withholding a reward (as, for example, in a timeout programme) from slipping into punishment. Much depends on the attitude of the staff.

Confidentiality

Confidentiality starts with the ideal that the patient's information is kept to the therapist and members of their team (on a need-to-know basis). However, information is about the family as well as about the child and the team membership may go wider than the immediate health staff. In particular, placements such as a special school can acquire an extraordinary insight into the family dynamics over time. The family's agreement must be negotiated for health staff to share information with the other agencies whether by mouth or through copy letters

Medication

There is increasing caution about the use of medication in minors and, while most of this is about its clinical effect, there are also legal qualms about treating someone who is not competent or even lacks the mental capacity, whether it is to give consent or to refuse. The legal distinctions are becoming better attuned to the shift from being a minor whose parents can give consent on their behalf, to being an adult for whom only the doctor or a court can authorise treatment (as being in their best interest).

Conclusion

The greater emphasis on, and skill in treating children in their own homes will increase the frequency and intensity of disturbance in those children who arrive in out-of-home placements. Increasing awareness of legal rights and concern about statutory demands will make responsible services more wary of providing care unless they are well supported by all the agencies available to the child. The management of disturbance is therefore a multiagency, multidisciplinary exercise.

Chapter 7

Disabled Children in Foster Care: A review of interventions that improve health outcomes for children and support carers

Thomas Kus and Heather Payne

Introduction

This chapter examines the evidence base for effective interventions for children doubly in need, in that they are both disabled and living away from home. Children in foster care have well-recognized health, social, educational and emotional needs, but still suffer from the 'inverse care law' and are less able to access services to reverse these inequalities. Children living away from home are particularly vulnerable to changes in their home environment, social interactions, rules and boundaries, family and school contacts. Adaptation difficulties are common, particularly with regard to family norms and expectations, and communication of 'unwritten rules' and the situation may be compounded by placement breakdown.

Children with disabilities have similar problems with health, social and educational deficits, invisibility to and poor access to services. The particular problems of disabled children in foster care merit specific attention because of the concurrence and magnification of these common difficulties.

Children with disabilities require a range of care services, which may include:

- respite care, also described as a planned series of short-term breaks (stays away from the family home);
- shared care (where the child lives part of the week with the family of origin and the rest of the time with a linked foster family or in a residential placement); or
- full-time placement in a foster family, residential home or school.

The primary need of the child is usually determined by the type of disability, but this may be accentuated or compounded by their social situation. Providers are often unaware what interventions are beneficial in meeting the often complex needs of disabled children in the care system. Effective service provision should be based on a multidisciplinary approach to the child and their disability, and promote special training and support for carers.

For practical reasons this review will mainly focus on children with physical disabilities, developmental delay and learning difficulties. The issue of short-term breaks as a means of providing support to families with disabled children who primarily live at home is a rather different problem and can only be mentioned briefly in the context of providing respite for foster carers themselves.

Background

The Children Act 1989 described disabled children and young people as those who are 'blind, deaf, or dumb or suffer from mental disorder of any kind or are substantially handicapped by illness, injury or congenital deformity' (Children Act 1989 Section 17/11), a definition taken (unchanged) from the National Assistance Act 1948 (Butler and Roberts 1997). Children with disabilities are also covered by the Disabled Persons Act 1986, which states that local authorities have a duty to 'provide welfare services to any persons within its area if this is necessary in order to meet the needs of that person' (Disabled Persons Act 1986 Sections 5 and 6). This includes the provision of special education services and the planning for transition to adult services where indicated (Department of Health (DH) 1991c). According to the Children Act Report 2001 by the end of 2001 social services in England and Wales were in touch with 29 700 disabled children and their families. However, for 40% of these children service provision was limited to intermittent short-term respite care (DH 2001).

People Like Us was a key document published by Sir William Utting in 1997. It provided a review of the situation of the UK care system following disclosures of serious and systematic abuse in Looked After children. It identified disabled children as particularly vulnerable and established important facts about their situation in care (Utting 1997: 79–88).

- Children with disabilities were found to be eight times more likely to be in care than non-disabled children and constituted 28% of all children in care.
- Evidence of physical or sexual abuse was found in 15% of disabled children.

Difficulties in communication and the understanding of limits between necessary care activities including intimate care and abuse underline the difficulties in protecting these children. It is important that children and their carers are able to communicate openly and that security measures and safeguards are in place to prevent abuse. These include appropriate staff vetting and training, regular inspections of care settings including specialist schools, educating children about their rights and promoting a high level of vigilance for all professionals involved in their care.

What do disabled children need?

In 1999 the UK Government initiated *Quality Protects* in England (www.dcsf.gov.uk/qualityprotects), a 5-year programme with a budget of £883 million aimed at improving the care for Looked After children (*Children First* in Wales (www.childrenfirst.wales.gov.uk)). It was based on the Utting Report (1997) and the publication of a consultation document *Promoting the Health of Looked After Children* (DH 1999) and the main recommendations for Looking After disabled children were as follows.

- 'Children with specific social needs arising out of disability should be living in families or appropriate settings in the community where their assessed needs are met and reviewed' (Council for Disabled Children 1999).
- Identification of special educational needs in children with disabilities: this is an important factor in the decision-making process as the needs of children with profound disabilities may be best met in a residential school placement.
- Detailed health assessment and care plan: this should be based on all available information and the role of the consultant community paediatrician in providing or coordinating this assessment is emphasized.
- Identification of barriers to successful integration into care placements: this involves looking at provisions needed in the care setting to enable disabled children to have sufficient opportunities for optimal development, social and community integration.
- Respite care: although this is mentioned in the context of short-term placements for children who usually live with their families it is also a major issue for those in long-term foster placements.
- Identification of the child's wishes and feelings: these should be identified and respected wherever possible and particular effort made to reduce communication barriers.

In a first report on the implementation of this programme a number of problems were identified with regards to Looked After children with disabilities (Council for Disabled Children 1999). These included different views on the definition of disability across agencies, lack of information and communication, partly due to uncertainties about confidentiality issues and incomplete information. The importance of clear protocols and multidisciplinary cross-agency working was highlighted as a major factor in overcoming these problems. Respite care issues were particularly highlighted for older children with autism and other challenging behaviours who are in foster care. It also found that schools were often underrepresented in the decision-making process even though many disabled children also have special educational needs. However, this was a very early report and despite the problems there was evidence that local management action plans were improving the outcomes for disabled children in care.

The special needs of disabled children in care

Many disabled children have complex needs that go beyond the traditional medical model of 'diagnose and treat'. Multidisciplinary working is a key factor in the successful implementation of individual care plans and this is even more important for disabled children in foster care who are particularly vulnerable. However, there are considerable practical difficulties in making multidisciplinary care plans work, often due to lack of communication and differences in set priorities and funding (Richardson et al 1989). Furthermore, neither child protection procedures nor foster/residential care systems were created with disabled children in mind and combining the two can be very challenging indeed.

The Carlile report refers to the increased needs for protection of children with disabilities (Carlile 2002 section 13.14:109). It emphasizes the importance of a team-based professional approach and specifically mentions the role of community nurses in this context.

George et al (1992) looked at the special educational needs of children in foster care and found that those needs were often not met because the provision of care for these children evolved around their need for protection. This American study did not look at disabled children in particular but it showed that simply providing a place of safety for children with special educational needs was not enough to ensure that they receive an education appropriate to their needs. These findings were confirmed in another case study of 12 randomly selected children with disabilities that found that even in cases where the responsible agencies had taken their special education needs into account there was still some dysfunction or disruption of services in 11 out of 12 children (Weinberg 1997). Whether this was due to difficulties in the special educational system in general or a result of being in care could not be answered by this study as it did not include a control group.

In the study by Robinson et al (1995) two models of care were compared for children under five: residential homes offering short-term accommodation and specialist day care services for under-fives. They found that both models worked well regarding outcome measures but there were problems with staff training and cooperation between agencies. It is worth noting that this study focused on the under-5s only and is therefore limited in its conclusions. Also, there is a general trend away from placements in residential homes, particularly for younger children, and some of the findings may not be easily transferable to foster care placements.

The special needs of carers for disabled children

In the past most disabled children were placed in residential homes where staff working patterns meant that care responsibilities were shared. However, there has been a recent trend towards more family-like placements in long-term foster placements, which have been shown to provide better opportunities for the individual development of disabled children than residential placements (Borthwick-Duffy et al 1992). A German study of 47 disabled children in care found that outcome parameters, such as the number of hospital admissions, behaviour problems, psychosomatic pain symptoms and enuresis were significantly less common in children living with foster families as compared with those in residential care homes (Weiler et al 1988).

The success of foster placements has also been demonstrated in a Dutch study looking at 78 children with learning difficulties and behaviour problems (Laan et al 2001). The Netherlands have introduced a system with an extensive matching and preparation period for both the child and the prospective family which precedes any decision about long-term placement:

- 74% of these children were still with the same family after 2 years or more, significantly more than the 58% who were placed as a 'crisis intervention' without prior matching;
- counselling and support were identified by 82% of foster carers as the main factors for successful placements;
- 80% stated that they were satisfied with the support they received.

Matching disabled children with prospective foster carers is a complex problem that requires careful consideration. Remaining within the existing local framework of school, health and voluntary services would usually be the best option for these children as it involves the least amount of disruption and makes contacts with the family easier. On the other hand, the availability of specialist foster placements is limited and meeting the needs of an individual child in the long term should be the deciding factor when considering the most suitable placement..

Finding a 'replacement family' has led to a move from residential to specialist foster care since the 1970s which has been shown to improve the outcomes for these children. The Finnish experience (Szymanski et al 1995) is that most children (and even adults) with disabilities or learning difficulties are in the care of professional foster carers who are paid a professional fee for their services. Perhaps this is the reason why there is no shortage of potential carers, which makes it easier to find the most suitable and thus the most likely successful foster placement for a disabled child.

In a recently published study Sinclair and Wilson (2003) looked at factors that may help to predict successful foster placements. They reviewed 596 foster placements across 7 representative boroughs across the UK. Although not specifically focused on children with disabilities, placements were more likely to be successful where:

- carers had good parenting skills;
- interacted well with the child; and
- were able to provide stability and an emotional bond.

The importance of having foster carers who are accurately selected, well trained and supported is again underlined in this study as the key for successful placements.

Many parents of non-disabled children can rely on extended family to provide periods of respite care and this is often a positive experience for all involved. Disabled children frequently require specialist care or may have behaviour problems that make the provision of respite by family members much more difficult. This is an even greater problem for disabled children in foster care although the mostly positive effects are clearly evident (Oswin 1991).

Challenging behaviour is a particularly common problem that often leads to the breakdown of foster placements. Pithouse et al (2002) investigated whether specific behaviour management training would improve outcomes for foster placements. In this randomized controlled study of 103 placements 53 were assigned to the training group and 53 to the control group. Although over 90% of carers found the training useful there were no significant outcome differences between the groups.

Cowen et al (2002) looked at 148 families and their 265 developmentally disabled children and found that:

- the parental stress index was significantly higher than in families of non-disabled children;
- a younger mother's age and negative health status were both significantly correlated with higher stress scores;
- respite care was shown to significantly reduce parental stress, parental depression, social isolation and child demandingness.

However, it is worth noting that the intervention sample was self-selected and the comparison data taken from a national survey, which may have had an impact on the results.

Ames (1996) looked at the experiences of 23 birth children aged 8–20 years within foster families looking after children with learning disabilities. This qualitative study using group discussions and semi-structured interviews within a self-selected cohort gave a generally positive picture of family integration although some adolescent girls felt that they were expected to take up additional responsibilities leading to tensions within the home. There were also issues of sharing personal space and time as the fostered children in their care often had complex disabilities and needs.

Summary
Disabled children in foster care are a heterogeneous group with often complex and challenging problems. Although they have essentially the same needs as similarly affected children living with their families it is important to remember that the reasons for requiring foster care imply that there are often additional difficulties as a result of abuse or neglect within their original environment. Furthermore the process of moving into foster care is often traumatic and involves significant changes which can be very difficult for disabled children.

The evidence indicates that successful outcomes for these children depend on a detailed, thorough assessment of their needs and the availability of well-matched, trained and supported specialist foster carers. National reviews and international examples show that good long-term outcomes are achievable and there are indications that the *Quality Protects* programme is leading to improvements in the care of disabled children.

Chapter 8

Education's Contribution to a Holistic Approach

Mike Searle and Allen Baynes

Introduction

It is often said that education is the best inoculation against social exclusion in later life. If that is true then no wonder so many children who enter the care system go on to such poor social and economic outcomes in later life. The education experience of too many children in care is a poor one when compared with their peers who stay out of the care system.

The education of children and young people in care is frequently characterized by a fragmented and discontinuous experience of school, leading to gaps in knowledge and skills. These gaps dramatically impact on attainment and lead to the development of attitudes and behaviour which can place them at odds with the discipline and behaviour policies in school. That in turn leads to this vulnerable group being excluded, either fixed term or permanently, for long periods from the very system which will best equip them to be included within society. It is a perverse irony that children and young people in care often fail in the schools that are run by their corporate parent, the local authority.

Children who are in the care system but who also have significant special educational needs that require special school provision not only face the same barriers to inclusion as their mainstream peers, but they have the additional disadvantage of their disability and their potential education segregation to contend with.

Although they are hopefully less likely than their mainstream peers to face exclusion, the other obstacles posed by their disability and the schooling require a substantial effort by professionals to reduce and minimize the challenges. These are our children who require the very best of coordinated support that can be offered and must be included as part of the good work that is developing for children in care that is identified later in this chapter.

In the UK this poor picture of the education of Looked After children is a national one and has existed for a long time. The Utting report (1997) drew public attention to the continuing educational under-achievement of young people in care. The needs of Looked After children have traditionally been a low priority in the education arena. This has been exacerbated since the introduction of the Education Reform Act in 1988, where the emphasis on the standards agenda has created even more pressures and the increased likelihood of marginalization on this already vulnerable group. They have, along with other vulnerable groups, been forced to the margins as schools have been ever more conscious of their need to perform in the local and national league tables with a focus on the children who can 'support' that performance.

Happily, there are clear signs that this is starting to change, not least because if standards are to rise yet further then that can only be achieved if the standards of vulnerable groups, such as Looked After children, are raised. This shift in emphasis was initially lead by additional funding for Looked After children through the *Vulnerable Children Grant* (www.dcfs.gov.uk/exclusions/VULNERABLE_CHILDREN/VULNERABLE_CHILDREN.cfm) in education and *Quality Protects* (www.dcfs.gov.uk/qualityprotects) funding in social care. Also, the issue of outcomes for children and young people in public care has been raised by the recent publication of research and guidance:

- *Education of Young People in Public Care* (Department for Education and Skills (DfES)/Department of Health (DH) 2000);
- *A Better Education for Children in Care* (Social Exclusion Unit (SEU) 2003);
- *Breaking the Cycle* (SEU 2004).

All of this research and guidance has been given new emphasis in the *Every Child Matters* and *Every Child Matters: Change for Children* agenda (Department for Education and Skills (DfES) 2003 and 2004b, (see also DfES 2004c and d)). The Children Act 2004 and the new joint inspection regime (JAR – Joint Area Review) sees the clear duty for collaborative working between agencies to operate. This should ensure that local authorities have no option other than to adopt the shared responsibility and holistic response to the needs of children and young people in care that this chapter advocates. The *Narrowing the Gap* project jointly funded by the Department for Children, Schools and Families (DCSF), the Local Government Association (LGA) and the Improvement and Development agency (IDeA), which will report later in 2008, will provide renewed impetus to ensure that the educational needs of children in care become a key priority in improving outcomes for vulnerable children (see www.lga.gov.uk/lga/core/page.do?pageId=234484 and LGA, DCSF and IDeA forthcoming publication).

Outcomes
The long-term outcomes for children and young people in care are extremely poor. This is despite the fact that many children go into resource intensive placements both in and out of their local authority. Whilst many placements offer a quality residential placement it is often not matched by the kind of education experience which

helps them to regain lost ground in terms of their education. Even if they do have a good educational experience this can often be lost with the next change of placement.

It must be remembered that many children in care, particularly those in foster care, enjoy school and some go on to be very successful in later life. However, for far too many their experience of school and further education is depressingly poor and places them at significantly greater risk than their peers in terms of the quality of their future life.

A SEU report on children in care reported that:

> at any one time, around 60 000 children are in care and in 2001–02, 41% of children in care were aged 10 or under. Most, some 80%, entered care because of abuse or neglect or for family reasons, less than 10% enter care because of their own behaviour.
>
> *(SEU 2003)*

Of that 10%, it is not known how many have behavioural difficulties as a result of their parenting experience, but one can believe that this might be very high.

Throughout their school career many children in care underperform. In the key stage tests at 7, 11 and 14, in 2005 only 10.8% achieved 5 A*–C grades compared with the national average of 57.1%. In 2007 the peformance on the same measure for children in care had risen to 12.6% but the gap with the rest of the school population has grown even wider as the national average had risen to 62%.

Not surprisingly perhaps those leaving care are vulnerable to later social exclusion:

- less than 5% go to university;
- between a quarter and a third of rough sleepers were once in care;
- they are more than two and a half times more likely to be a teenage parent;
- around a quarter of adults in prison have an experience of being in care;
- in 2001–02 only 46% of care leavers were known to be in employment, education or training at age 19, compared with 86% of all 19-year-olds.

To fully understand the reasons for these woeful outcomes one probably has to have been in care: an experience that the overwhelming majority of teachers, social workers, other care professionals, politicians and policy planners can only guess at. The traumatic and negative psychological, social and emotional impact of being placed in care should not be underestimated, even when a child is being taken out of a real or potentially threatening environment.

The move into care when it happens can be very sudden with little time to say goodbye to parents, siblings or even the family pet, or to collect items of personal significance from the family home. This sudden emotional loss is bound up with a whole raft of other highly personal issues:

- Where am I going?
- Who will be there? Will I see my friends, family again?
- What have I done to make this happen?

If you have been lucky to have had a secure family upbringing it is difficult to imagine the trauma that exists around a move into care.

To be taken from your home, no matter how poor it has been, to have your limited worldly belongings often in a plastic bin bag and then to be taken to another often alien part of your area or in a different part of the country, is an event which will stay with you for the rest of your life. If this new placement is unsatisfactory or breaks down you then repeat the process. I wonder at what point you would start to lose your trust in adults in authority?

You might also, as part of the move, have to change schools with its new systems, new adults who know very little about you and to be potentially faced with the discontinuity in the curriculum, new peer group to integrate into and in which you carry the stigma and shame that accompanies being in care, etc. One can begin to see the challenge that children in care face even if what they are moving to is better than what they have left.

The challenge for professionals who work with Looked After children is to understand these potential consequences for children moving into care and to work together to minimize the trauma but also have in place positive systems to maximize the child's integration into their new placement. It is vital to listen to the child, to understand their needs and to ensure that whatever service that you provide is of high quality and fit for purpose.

National guidance

The last 20 years have seen the publication of a wide range of guidance on the inclusion of children and young people, in particular those who are in danger of social exclusion with a particular emphasis on those who are in public care. This guidance has raised awareness and underlined the need for action to ensure that all children achieve their potential. There has also been an emphasis on placing the responsibility for promoting the educational attainment of young people in care on to the local authority.

As noted previously the Utting Report (1997) underlined the poor performance of provision for children in care and identified education as the critical dimension of their 'welfare' as defined by the Children Act 1989.

The Department of Education and Employment (DfEE) Circulars 10/99 and 11/99 in July 1999, relating to social inclusion pupil support identified Looked After children as a key vulnerable group and went on to tighten procedures relating to attendance and exclusion as well as setting out the need for all children to be in full-time (up to 25 hours) appropriate education.

These publications were quickly followed by joint DfES/DH guidance in 2000, *Education of Young People in Public Care*. This valuable guidance has prompted much of the recent improvement in the education of children in care. The guidance promoted the development of better corporate parenting, the importance of education to this group and introduced the use of *Personal Education Plans* (PEP) on a national scale. Underpinning this guidance was the importance of having good information on the child, as any parent would have and using this information together with the support of other relevant agencies to improve the provision and support to the child or young person.

In September 2003 the SEU produced its recommendation on how best to raise the educational attainment of children in care in: *A Better Education for Children in Care*. This report identified five key reasons why children in care underachieve in education.

- **Instability**: although most children who enter care do so once and only have one care placement, 1 in 7 had three or more care placements in 2001–2002 and over a third of the young people consulted as part of the report had changed school twice as a result of a change in care placement.

- **Time out in school**: a significant minority of children in care are in non-mainstream settings with some receiving only a few hours of tuition per week. Many miss long periods of education because they do not have a school place; they are excluded or their attendance is poor.

- **Help with school work**: many children in care need extra support in education, either because they have missed key areas of curriculum, or because they have special educational needs which may be attributable, at least in part, to the fragmented or discontinuous nature of their education.

- **Support and encouragement**: it is important that carers and social workers supporting children's education should have high expectations for their children, a clear understanding of their roles and responsibilities, up-to-date information about education, and the skills to support development and learning. This area also includes the support and encouragement for out of school and youth work activities that is so important for children's wider learning and development. The expectation being that children in care need the same support and encouragement that children in stable, secure and loving homes receive.

- **Health and well-being**: a child's emotional, mental and physical health strongly influence educational outcomes. As noted previously placement moves can exacerbate health problems, make diagnosis harder and leave children exposed to bullying and trauma. School can boost a child's health through raising self-confidence, self-esteem and enable participation in sports and leisure activities as well as giving access to health education.

The government green paper *Every Child Matters* (DfES 2003) was published in the same month as the SEU report in 2003 and has lead to unprecedented change in the way services are going to be delivered for children. The green paper, which was a response to Lord Laming's report on the death of Victoria Climbie, proposed a step change in the way government, both local and national, will meet the needs of *all* children and young people.

Every Child Matters (DfES 2003) evolved into the *Every Child Matters: Change for Children* (DfES 2004b) agenda which has the Children Act 2004 at its centre. This puts a duty on all those working with children, the children's workforce, to work collaboratively and to share information to help deliver better services for children.

This better service is characterized by an emphasis on five key outcomes, drawn up after widespread consultation with children, young people and their families. The five outcomes are:

- enjoying and achieving;
- making a positive contribution;
- being healthy;
- staying safe;
- economic well-being.

These five outcomes have been established to set a marker to help all children to achieve their potential. The challenge is for the children's workforce, whether in education, health, social care or the voluntary sector to work together to ensure that these outcomes are genuinely open to all children particularly those in vulnerable groups such as children in care.

Positive practical action

The five outcomes from the *Change for Children* agenda offer a framework for developing support for Looked After children that all agencies working with children and young people should recognize and support. It is a framework that was developed through wide consultation with stakeholders including children and has been well received by professionals across the sector.

Telford and Wrekin had the early benefit of being a pilot Children's Trust and a Pathfinder for IRT (Information Referral and Tracking), now ISA (Information Sharing and Assessment). These two initiatives helped move forward what was already good collaborative working practice across education, health and social care. The authority has adopted the five outcomes as a way of developing multiagency working and strategic planning and this model was adopted to help plan outcomes for Looked After children under the acronym HOPSLAC (Holistic Planning and Support for Looked After Children) see Figure 8.1.

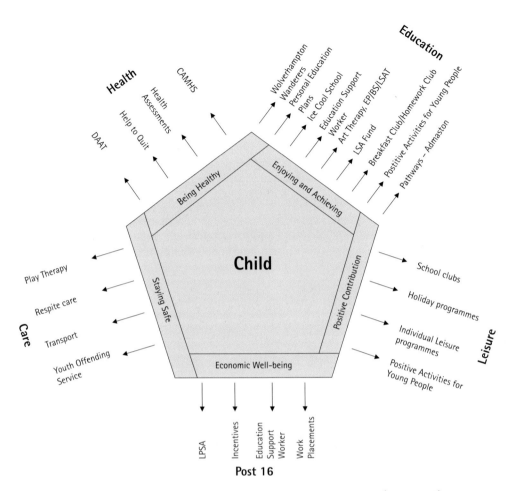

Figure 8.1 Holistic Planning and Support for Looked After Children (HOPSLAC). Admaston, shared placement unit for primary aged student with behavioural difficulties; BS, behaviour support; CAMHS, child and adolescent mental health services; DAAT, drug and alcohol action team; EP, educational psychologist; LPSA, local public service agreements; LSA, local service agreement; LSAT, learning support advisory teacher.

From some time before the publication of *Every Child Matters* (2003), Telford and Wrekin recognized that improving outcomes for children in public care was a high priority for the local authority and was not the responsibility of any one agency. It was a joint responsibility across the local authority and its key partner agencies of health, police and the voluntary sector. With the support of the pilot Children's Trust initiative the local partnership board was strengthened to form a Children's and Young People's Strategic Partnership Board (CYPSPB). This board is well supported by elected members who understand the term corporate parenting and its attendant responsibilities and their importance as locally elected representatives in supporting the outcomes for children in their authority's care.

The CYPSPB oversees the strategic planning that is driving the operational delivery of support and intervention to positively impact on children in care. Importantly, children and young people, including those who are in care, have a direct voice into the strategic board through the young people's forum. This broad representative group are consulted on policy development and many of the initiatives described in this chapter are shaped, or have been developed in collaboration with the young people themselves. Their views have been fundamental to any success that has been achieved. It is a key part of the corporate parenting manager's role, and that of the team, to listen to what young people say about the support that is offered to them and to encourage them to identify better ways of delivering that support. The notion of listening to the children themselves is becoming an integral way of service development and delivery across Telford and Wrekin. This has been supported by excellent initiatives developed through the Children's Fund, a key one being the funding of the 'Leisure and Fun Coordinator' who has specific responsibility for developing out of school support for Looked After children.

One of the key elements in all of the initiatives that have been developed for vulnerable children is the notion that staff should be 'champions for children'. This does not just mean front line workers who have a direct input with the children but also corporate directors in health, education, social care through to paediatricians, teachers, youth workers.

This broad strategic planning framework provided by CYPSPB, together with the national advice and guidance, and underpinned by the ideas, thoughts and aspirations of our young people and the empowerment of key staff as champions is starting to change how the authority makes provision for its vulnerable children. There is however, a huge amount of work to be done as the wealth of anecdotal good news needs to be consolidated into outcome measures that significantly narrow the attainment and achievement gap between vulnerable children and their peers.

As Figure 8.1 shows there are a range of activities that support the attainment of the five key outcomes.

Enjoying and achieving
The key to achieving these outcomes is ensuring that Looked After children are in education and are supported to achieve their potential. This is not easy given the difficulties already noted that frequently accompany a move into care. The best place for most Looked After children to achieve this is in a mainstream school. To support this we have ensured that every school has a *designated teacher for children in care*, this is relatively easy as most schools although wary of added bureaucracy, are keen to be supportive. The next stage is to offer all the designated teachers training and importantly this should be joint training with social care staff. The training needs to set out the shared agenda between social care and education, develop the understanding of the needs of children in care to enable them to succeed in education and ensure there is a growth in understanding of the barriers to education and how they can be removed.

The designated teacher's role is unusual in that some schools have very little contact with Looked After children whilst for others it is a part of everyday school life. The designated teacher's role is to be that advocate for Looked After children within their school, to raise staff awareness of pupils' needs and to ensure that all of these children have a personal education plan. They must also ensure that this group of children benefit from access to the wider school curriculum and that they have the opportunity to participate in cultural, leisure and sporting activity within the school. The designated teacher should be the focal point for support for other agencies who are charged with meeting the needs of Looked After children.

To help Looked After children's needs to be identified and met all children in public care should have a personal education plan (PEP) (DfES/DH 2000, paragraphs 5.16–5.26). It is the responsibility of the child's social worker to inform the school and initiate the PEP. However, the school can provide a key focal point of the multiagency planning and support that will provide the 'team around the child'.

The PEP provides an opportunity to promote education as a priority for the child among the significant adults involved with the child. A key element of any PEP should be input from the child such as worries, ambitions and ideas for reaching targets. This element of the PEP provides a useful format for developing an ongoing dialogue with the child in relation to their education and aspirations and can be used by teachers or social care staff.

The PEP should cover the following areas:

- an achievement record;
- developmental and educational needs;
- short-term targets;
- long-term plans and aspirations.

The good work in the PEP can easily be lost if pupils move placement and the designated teacher should ensure that the current PEP is forwarded to the next education placement.

Best practice and government guidelines say that the PEP should be agreed within 20 days of the child being Looked After by the local authority or joining a new school and that it should be reviewed concurrently with the care plan i.e. within 28 days, 3 months and then at least every 6 months. As with all children points of transition between key stages, particularly between Key Stage 2 and 3 (secondary transfer) are crucial and the time when joint planning and sharing of information are essential to maintain a child's positive experience of education.

Not all children because of their experiences prior to and after entry into the care system are able to access full-time mainstream education. It is therefore essential that there are well thought out and meaningful alternatives to education which provide a supported ladder or stepping stone back into school. This provision often needs only to be short term in nature while the young person comes to terms with or resolves trauma or upheaval in their home life. These settings can provide a highly supportive and therapeutic environment which school cannot hope to match in the busy context in which they operate.

In Telford we have set up alternative provision at a study centre at the local ice rink. The 'Ice Cool School' as it is known provides a high staff to pupil ratio with access to a wide range of learning materials, often provided through the information and communication technology infrastructure available in Telford and Wrekin. We have also worked with the study support provision available at Wolverhampton Wanderers Football Club to provide football coaching linked to a GNVQ in sports and leisure. The coaching has proved to be highly motivating to pupils whose attendance has gone from 40% to well over 90%. So successful have these provisions been for vulnerable children, we are now working with our local football club AFC Telford to develop a non-league study support centre to premiership standards. This has gone on to be recognized as an example of national good practice.

We hope that this venture will provide a highly motivating and appropriate venue to support the young people at Key Stage 4 in getting qualifications, raise their self-esteem and provide them with the motivation to access careers in the local leisure and recreation industry. This local venture has the support of the local further education college which is less than 100 metres from the football ground so enhancing opportunities to move into further education once the young people leave school. The collaborative work between the local authority, AFC Telford, the further education college and the Football Association will make this a success and provide a template for other alternative provision that is needed.

Positive contribution
The close links that have been developed with partner agencies have been enhanced by the role of the 'Leisure and Fun Coordinator'. Working as part of the 'Corporate Parenting Team' she has helped develop a wide range of activities which have positively engaged young people and in so doing has enabled them to make a positive contribution to the work of the authority and in support of their peers who are in care.

The coordinator post has been funded through the Children's Fund and was a post created in response to the request of the Looked After children to have someone to organize clubs for them. As well as setting up a range of clubs and activities ranging from a poetry club to horse riding and football, the coordinator has proved to be a powerful female role model.

The clubs have had a demonstrable effect on the children's self-esteem and when part of a package with the Ice Cool School or football project this has led to children maintaining their residential and educational placement as well as supporting a return to home for a number of children.

The coordinator along with other members of the corporate parenting team have organized with PGL (a provider of activity courses and holidays) a summer camp for the last two years enabling Looked After youngsters to have a week at one of their camps. The children have experienced a wide range of outdoor activities such as canoeing, raft building, climbing, adventure trails and mountain biking. These summer camps have not only helped placement stability by ensuring carers have respite, they have given the young people the chance to experience success at activities they would not normally have access to.

Another innovative activity was a Key Stage 3 revision/homework club. This involved an hour's supported revision/homework followed by a remote controlled car club. The young people did their homework then played with the cars and if they attended every session they got to keep the car. Not surprisingly attendance for the homework club was very high.

In turn the young people have given back to the authority:

● by being willing members of consultative groups;
● by being participants in the interviewing process for a number of posts;
● by being co-presenters and organizers of the annual awards evening for Looked After children; and
● five of our children have received national awards for their commitment and involvement in the activities set up by the corporate parenting team.

Being healthy
The health of Looked After children, like their education experience, has been some way below that which you would want for your child. A key part of the problem is that health has too often been seen as a separate area and the notion that good health is part of other aspects of a child's life, like leisure activities and diet has not been fully appreciated.

The greater engagement of the children in school, alternative education schemes and in the clubs and wider activities has had a very positive impact on their self-esteem and the children's wider mental health. This and the increased range of adults who are taking an active interest in the children and what is being done for them has raised their feelings of self-worth and increased their expectations and knowledge of their rights. This is enabling these young people to be both more assertive and conscious of the need for health support to help them gain the most from life.

All Looked After children now have access to a dedicated sexual health worker and to the drug and alcohol abuse teams. They are now a targeted group within all health promotion activities and there is now the infrastructure around the children to capitalize on and reinforce the benefits of these opportunities.

The whole system of health assessments is under review and in future there will be an emphasis on making these community based and more user friendly both in terms of the assessment and the bureaucracy that surrounds the assessment.

Staying safe
Staying safe is in many ways the cornerstone of all the provision that we make for the children. Many of these children are accommodated because of concerns for their safety. All of the positive activities and experiences that we give these young people raises these expectations, self-esteem and their ability to be assertive about who they are and what they want from life. This contributes to their personal safety now and in the future. Their raised profile across the authority means that their needs are known to community safety and other council activities such as transport which impact on their safety.

The key people in keeping children safe are their foster carers and residential social workers and it is recognized that we need a energetic, well-resourced and well-trained team of foster carers who have swift access to professional support and advice and to respite care. This is a major challenge to all authorities but one which is now at the top of our agenda.

Economic well-being
This outcome is arguably the most important to young people in care because of the impact it will have on their future life and, as has already been noted, the statistics indicate over representation of care leavers in many negative areas of life such as rough sleepers and drug use. It is also the outcome in which support reduces, often very rapidly, as the young people become care leavers.

There are a number of key factors which influence whether a young person goes onto further/higher education or whether they go into the workplace or onto benefits. Clearly their experience of education has too often been a negative one that has impacted on the pupil's self-esteem and the value that they place on education. To overcome this pupils, particularly those not in foster care, require a significant level of support at Key Stage 4 to ensure that they attend school, that they are supported with coursework and homework and that they are entered for and attend exams. Even if a young person is not fully engaged with education you can, with targeted support, ensure that they do achieve external examination success. The support teacher and support worker for Looked After children in Telford and Wrekin focus their efforts on engaging and re-engaging young people in education. They have developed targeted subject support which maximizes the young people's attainment and through the positive relationships that they develop with the young people have encouraged the majority, (over 90%), of the Looked After pupils to stay on into further education. There are significant issues around sustaining that further education placement and so a Connexions worker is now part of the corporate parenting team to ensure that support is offered throughout the leaving care process.

However, local authorities including Telford and Wrekin can do much more. There are now many examples of councils developing their own work experience schemes and guaranteeing employment within the council for care leavers. After all, as already noted, the council is often the biggest family firm in the area.

Conclusion

We can see that there are many things that have been achieved to improve the education experience of children in care and we can see that it is not just education on its own that is required. It is about the whole child and it is about raising their aspirations, their expectations and their feelings of self-worth and this can only be truly achieved by listening and engaging the children and young people themselves. Once you have that there is no limit to what can be achieved.

To do this however, the local authority, together with partner agencies particularly health, needs to ensure that all children in care at whatever age should experience quality collaborative support and provision so that all the young persons needs are identified and met wherever possible. They have to act like any good parent would. However, given the level of need that children and young people in care have, perhaps we should raise our demands and not settle for just being a good corporate parent but our aim should be to be a 'super' corporate parent. After all these are our children and young people.

Chapter 9
Finding Out What Disabled Children with Communication Impairments Want

Catherine Baines

Introduction

A group of young people with communication impairments told researchers these are some of the things that really annoy them:

- they don't wait for me to finish what I've got to say – it takes longer for me to use my communication book than if I was using speech;
- they pretend they understand what I've said;
- they finish my sentences for me without asking me whether that is OK – sometimes it's OK sometimes it's not but they should ask me;
- they talk to the person who is with me and not to me;
- they ask me more than one question at a time;
- they act as if I'm 6 months old. (from Morris 2002)

Disabled children living away from home have the same rights as other children living away from home to tell people what they want.

Some disabled children who have severe visual or hearing difficulties but are of average intelligence may have some difficulty telling people what they want. Children with severe visual impairments and average intelligence will be able to express themselves orally, though they need help to communicate in writing. Children with severe hearing loss and average intelligence will have difficulty expressing themselves orally and being understood, but usually they will have learnt to use British sign language from a young age. But, it will be more difficult for disabled children with high support needs. These children will typically have little or no speech, a limited capacity to understand what is said to them and other physical and learning disabilities and it will be difficult for them to express their views clearly and be understood. Finding out what these children want calls for people working with them also to understand the meaning of facial expressions, gestures and body language that they will use to express their wishes and feelings. Some may also use communication aids.

All disabled children with communication impairments but particularly those with severe impairments should be given all the help and support they need so that they can communicate effectively. For them to achieve effective communication is one of the keys to improving the quality of these children's lives.

Looked After disabled children and young people with high support needs are more likely to be placed in a residential institution than other types of Looked After children. They are less likely to be placed with foster parents. Disabled children who are not Looked After but are sent away from home for their education tend to go away to school at a younger age; many are placed in residential schools a long way from their families. It is essential that those involved in the decision to send a child away from home and the staff in the residential setting where they will be living pay attention to how that child communicates and the amount and type of help they need to tell people what they want.

This chapter focuses on disabled children in residential settings – usually residential schools – and not those placed with foster parents. Some are likely to be in 52-week placements. It addresses the challenges facing people working with children with severe communication impairments.

Messages in policy documents

Since the 1980s policy guidance from the Government has said that all children and young people including those living away from home should be involved in decisions affecting them and their views should be taken into account. Since the mid-1990s policy makers at national and local level have also sought to involve children and young people in discussions on new policy ideas and changes in the way services are provided.

Below are the main policy documents issued by the Government in recent years that include material about disabled children or those with special educational needs.

- *The Special Educational Needs Code of Practice* (Department for Education and Skills (DfES) 2001): 'Children and young people with special educational needs have a unique knowledge of their own needs and circumstances and *their own views* about what sort of help they would like to help them make the most of their education' (emphasis added, paragraph 3.2) and 'Pupils' views should be sought and recorded as part of the statutory review process where possible, as well as within the IEP [Individual Education Plan] and any other assessment and review' (paragraph 3.15).
- The Commission for Social Care Inspection's *Residential Special Schools: National Minimum Standards. Inspection Regulations* (DH 2002b): standard 2 states 'Children's opinions, and those of their families or significant others, are sought

over key decisions which are likely to affect their daily life and their future. Feedback is given following consultations.' Paragraph 2.5 refers to 'the school providing frequent and suitable means for any child, *using their preferred method of communication* to make their wishes and feelings known regarding their care and treatment. . .' (emphasis added).

- *Removing Barriers to Achievement: The Government's Strategy for SEN* (DfES 2004e): chapter 3 refers to 'all children [having] a right to have their views taken into account in decisions about their education.' This chapter notes that 'involving them in decision-making enriches their learning and helps them develop life-skills such as problem solving and negotiation.' It recognizes that 'all children, even those with the most severe or complex needs, will have views about their education and the choices before them, and all should be enabled to communicate their wishes, using specialist tools and techniques where appropriate'.

- *The National Service Framework for Children, Young People and Maternity* (DH 2004a): standard 11 says children and young people and their families should be actively involved in all decisions affecting them and in shaping local services. It stresses the need for professionals to 'ensure that disabled children, especially children with high communication needs, are not excluded from the decision-making process' and to 'consider the needs of children who rely on communication equipment or who use non-verbal communication such as sign language.'

While none of these documents is specifically setting out policies for disabled children living away from home, the policy message about making sure that children can say what they want to say, and have their wishes and feelings taken into account, is as much addressed to people working in that area, as to people working with disabled and non-disabled children living at home.

Messages from research

Some of the research into disabled children living away from home looks at how disabled children with communication impairments express their views. The key message from the studies described below is that, on the whole, people working with disabled children and people making decisions about services for them do not routinely ensure that the children's views are heard. This is especially the case with children with communication impairments who live away from home.

People Like Us: The Report of the Review of the Safeguards for Children Living Away from Home (Utting 1997) said children with communication difficulties needed help to tell people they are being ill treated. It recommended more work on how to communicate with such children including developing non-verbal means of communication. *The Government Response to the Children's Safeguards Review* (UK government 1998) said the Council for Disabled Children and Triangle had been commissioned to provide a list of resources available to help practitioners communicate more effectively with disabled children.

Still Missing? (Morris 1998) reported on a study of three local authority social services departments and how they were implementing the Children Act 1989 as it applied to disabled children. This found:

- little evidence that disabled children's wishes and feelings about their placements were being sought. Typically the child's view section of the assessment form was left blank or had comments like 'she is unable to verbally communicate';
- parents were relied on to represent the views of older children when the social worker felt the level of impairment prohibited communication between him or her and the child;
- the majority of disabled children in contact with social services departments had communication impairments;
- social workers rarely had specialist training to help them communicate with the children.

Disabled Children and Residential Schools: A Survey of Local Authority Policy and Practice (Abbott et al 2000) looked at how 21 local authorities made decisions about disabled children going to residential schools. This found:

- education departments rarely sought views from the children;
- while social services departments were better at doing this, they tended just to ask children who could communicate. They used phrases in their reports like a child's 'inability' to communicate;
- the decision-making process tended to be dominated by other issues so that it was all too easy for the children's views to be lost.

On the other hand, the research also noted that authorities that had carried out pilot or development projects which included the views of children reported they had found out things about the children that they had not known before.

The Best Place to be? (Abbott et al 2001) examined the circumstances in which disabled children and young people were sent to residential schools in four local authorities. The research included semi-structured interviews with 18 children and observations and discussions with a key worker or teacher of 14 other children whose level of learning difficulty meant a semi-structured interview would not work. The research found:

- some children felt they had been involved in the decision;
- some parents said it was not possible to involve the child in the discussion about the decision because of the level of impairment;
- education and social work professionals did little to communicate with children with no speech. One educational psychologist said 'Ideally. . .they would want to meet the child [but] the approach is different if the child does not communicate verbally. . . [they] tend to rely on staff. . .and on parents. . .'. Social workers said lack of time prevented them building up a relationship with a child in a residential school, especially if the child had a communication impairment.

The report also contains material collected by the researchers that shows children with communication impairments can express themselves clearly and effectively.

Care and Treatment? Supporting Children with Complex Needs in Healthcare Settings (Stalker et al 2003) looked at the circumstances of 15 children in a variety of settings in England and Scotland. It found:

- no settings had procedures for routinely consulting children and young people especially those with communication impairments;
- children in medical wards felt they had more say and choice in their day to day lives though their wishes were not always acted upon;
- children in a residential school had less say, because staff thought their level of learning disability made it difficult for them to make choices;
- young people in a learning disability hospital were not involved in discussions about future placements because staff thought they would not be able to cope with the uncertainty inherent in such discussions.

Your Shout! A Survey of the Views of 706 Children and Young People in the Public Care (Timms and Thorburn 2003) summarizes responses to a questionnaire sent out via the Who Cares? Trust. Two of its key themes were: experience of decision making in court and participation in care plans. Responses came from a self-selected group, so the information obtained cannot be taken as representative. Only 12% of the respondents (81 young people) said they had either a disability or long-term health problem. The response to the survey suggested disability made no difference to what the children and young people said about participation in decision making. Of the respondents 43% felt they were listened to and 27% did not know. In the case of court decisions the survey found mixed messages about whether children felt they could express their views and expect them to be taken into account.

"It Doesn't Happen to Disabled Children": Child Protection and Disabled Children (National Working Group on Child Protection and Disability 2003) states that disabled children often lack access to the help they need with communication. Communication systems often lack the language necessary to disclose abuse, making it difficult for disabled children to find an appropriate vocabulary to tell others about what is happening to them. This report draws attention to the common failure to consult disabled children about their experiences, views, wishes and feelings. It also notes that disabled children in general had little choice and control over many aspects of their lives.

Progress on Safeguards for Children Living Away from Home: A Review of Action since the People Like Us Report (Stuart and Baines 2004b) found that in general children and young people were much more involved in discussions about policy issues, though they were still not sufficiently involved in decisions affecting their own lives. It commented that children were still not being listened to or involved in decision making and policy development in some settings including health settings, particularly where children have complex needs and/or spend a long time as inpatients. There was scope for improving training in the communication skills people needed when working with children and young people including with disabled children and young people. 'Authorities and organisations need to ensure that their staff have enough *time* to communicate properly with children and young people, particularly those who are disabled. . .' (emphasis added). The companion document *Safeguards for Vulnerable Children: Three Studies on Abusers, Disabled Children and Children in Prison* (Stuart and Baines 2004a) noted that the criminal justice system was still failing to prosecute those who had abused disabled children and that 'help with communication difficulties was essential' to help children give evidence.

Importance of hearing the views of disabled children

Internationally and nationally it has long been taken as the norm that all children and young people should be:

- actively involved in all decisions affecting them;
- able to say what they think, have their views listened to and taken into account.

Articles 12 and 13 in the UN Convention of the Rights of the Child (www.unicef.org.uk/tz/rights/convention.asp) (ratified by the UK Government in 1991) says that States Parties must ensure all children have the right to freedom of expression 'in all matters affecting the child' and 'the right shall include freedom to seek, receive and impart information and ideas of all kinds'. Article 23 says that States Parties should 'recognise that a mentally or physically disabled child should enjoy a full and decent life. . .[States Parties] should facilitate the child's active participation in the community.'

In *"It Doesn't Happen to Disabled Children"* (National Working Group on Child Protection and Disability 2003) contributors Ruth Marchant and Marcus Page from Triangle, in arguing for a rights-based approach to providing services for disabled children, say that the right to communication is one of three basic human rights for disabled children. This right sits with the right to safety and the right to express one's feelings and have these taken into account. While this concept is recognized in the Children Act 1989 and guidance issued by government departments, this rights-based approach is not yet found in all settings attended by disabled children, especially in residential settings. Disabled children with communication impairments living away from home are less likely to be helped to communicate their views and say what they want. They may also not be helped to take part in discussions about the decision to send them away from home. So this group of children are being denied a right that other children can and do exercise freely.

Disabled children and young people themselves say that 'they want to be listened to when decisions are made about their lives' (DH 2004a). Ruth Marchant and Marcus Page (National Working Group on Child Protection and Disability 2003) acknowledge that helping disabled children with communication impairments to exercise their right to communication is not easy and presents challenges to everyone involved. But people working with such children and young people are failing to provide the right help and support, if they do not strive to make sure such children are given the opportunity to say what they think about things and to have their views taken into account.

What prevents disabled children and young people from communicating effectively?

There are a number of barriers that, in combination, prevent this group of disabled children and young people from communicating effectively. The starting point is a failure by society as a whole to recognize that disabled children with communication impairments are children first and should be afforded the same opportunities as all children. This results in a failure to recognize that such children have the same right as other children to communicate their views, feelings and ideas and say what they want to say. In order to exercise this right they have to overcome the following hurdles.

- An assumption that disabled children with communication impairments cannot meaningfully express themselves and take part in decisions affecting their lives. While it is more difficult for these children to communicate clearly and unambiguously, it is possible to help them do this. Social workers should not record in an assessment form that the child 'is unable to communicate'. Not trying to support these children's efforts to say what they want or feel will result in them becoming angry, frustrated, withdrawn and un-cooperative, and switching off from their surroundings. This makes it more difficult for people to work with such children.

- A failure to recognize the importance of helping children with communication impairments to communicate their wishes and feelings. This could be construed as a form of discrimination. If these children are not being supported to say what they want, they are being denied one of the rights available to other children. It implies that the views of such children are not important when it comes to making decisions about things like what they feel about going away from home. It also implies that they cannot exercise any sort of choice.

- A failure to recognize that disabled children with communication impairments need much more time in order to express their views, and staff working with such children need to spend a lot of time getting to know how the child communicates. This is a fundamental problem that has to be solved if these children are to be helped to communicate effectively. A rights-based approach to providing help and support for this group would do much to ensure policy makers and senior managers enabled front line staff to have enough time to allow a disabled child with a communication impairment to say what they wanted, and play a full part in discussions about going away from home and in reviews when they are away from home.

- Making sure that any communication aid used by the child is available and in working order in *all* settings they attend. This is a factor for all disabled children with communication impairments, but it is particularly important for children living away from home. Staff in the school or other institution need to know how the aid works and how to get it repaired when or if it breaks down.

- Lack of knowledge and understanding about the different communication aids and methods now available. It is time consuming to research this, but it is essential to find out as much as possible in order to help and support the child to communicate effectively. The next section lists some of the sources of advice about materials etc available for practitioners.

- Inadequate training of staff in how to use different communication methods effectively. This is important for front line staff as well as other professionals who see the child occasionally. The research shows that staff dealing with disabled children already recognize the importance of being trained to use different communication methods, so that they can support such children's efforts to communicate their wishes and feelings.

- Some communication aids do not have some important words or meanings in them. Some do not have words, symbols or signs about private parts of the body. This means that a disabled child who is being or has been abused cannot explain this and be properly understood. This can result in disabled children who use communication aids not being given adequate protection from abuse.

- Disabled children living with their families also face these hurdles, but not to the same extent, and their parents or main carers will be there to help them overcome some of them. Disabled children with communication impairments who live away from home do not have easy access to their families, so the staff in residential schools or children's homes need to do more to ensure they can communicate effectively.

More needs to be done to enable all disabled children with communication impairments including those living away from home, to say what they want. Education and social work professionals know that it takes a lot of time to communicate effectively with disabled children with communication impairments and that they need training to do this well. There is a long way to go before disabled children with communication impairments receive the appropriate help and support so that they can say what they want and have their wishes and feelings taken into account.

Getting to know how someone communicates and finding out their views

This section looks at what is involved in finding out what the child wants before they go away to school, what is likely to help them communicate with the staff and other children in the residential school and lists sources of practical advice.

Planning to send a disabled child to a residential school has to include attention to how the child communicates as part of that process. The conditions under which any child is sent to a residential school paid for out of the public purse should be set out in a contract between the funding authority and the school. The contract should be supported by a plan agreed by all parties – the parents, the child, the school and the funding authorities. The plan should include a *communication plan* to sit alongside the care plan (in the case of a Looked After child), the Individual Education Plan (IEP) and a contact plan to enable the child and the family to keep in touch with each other. A disabled child with communication impairments will also be helped if they have with them a *personal communication passport* to explain who they are, how they communicate their feelings, what different gestures and expressions mean, the important people in their life, and their likes and dislikes.

Preparing a communication plan

This will involve pooling all the information about how the child communicates, what different facial expressions, gestures etc mean, what sort of help or training they have had in the past, what has been done to improve their capacity to communicate their wishes and feelings, any use of communication aids etc. As it is likely that some of this information is not written down, it will take time to draw up the plan and require discussions with the important people in the child's life including the child themselves and their family. The plan covering all the things listed above should be drawn up in consultation with the child and the family and reviewed along with the other plans for the child. The school should be sent a copy of the plan along with all the other documentation about the child.

Personal communication passport

CALL (Communication Aids for Language and Learning)[1] developed this concept to enable a disabled child with communication difficulties to tell other people not everything they know but the things that other people need to know about them. Gretel McEwen, a speech therapist and counsellor at the Community Learning Disabilities Team in Newcastle and Sally Miller, research communication therapist with the CALL centre in a paper presented at a study day in December 1993 wrote:

> The idea. . .is essentially a very simple one. The purpose is to provide a wholly personalized form of practical information about a person with communication difficulties who is unable to 'tell their own story' in order to help them, their family and staff. The Passport for each person will have a different format and emphasis, to reflect their own personal biography and their personal style and needs. A passport may be viewed as part of a 'total communication' approach or as a supplement to existing forms of augmentative communication used by the client.

Disabled children with communication impairments who are going away from home will find a personal communication passport an excellent tool for helping them share information about themselves with staff in their new school and the other children there. Other children when they go away from home to school can tell staff about their families, the people at home who are important to them, their likes and dislikes and so on. A personal communication passport serves the same purpose. The process of creating one is also valuable. It is likely to be a vehicle for enabling key people involved in the child's life to understand clearly what things matter to them, change the way they

---

1   The CALL centre, University of Edinburgh, Paterson's Land, Holyrood Road, Edinburgh EH8 8AQ
     Tel 0131 651 6235/6236

are seen as a person, and suggest new ways to find solutions about communication problems. The finished document will provide:

- practical functional information;
- consistency;
- continuity;
- increased confidence and sense of self-worth in the child.

The CALL website (http://www.callcentrescotland.org.uk) provides a template for creating a personal communication passport. This suggests that its pages should cover these topics:

- all about me;
- you need to know;
- my family;
- my friends;
- special people;
- special things;
- things I like to talk about;
- how I communicate;
- you can help me communicate;
- fun things I like to do;
- places I like going;
- things I don't like;
- I'm working on this. . .;
- Help!
- eating and drinking;
- what's my eyesight like.

There are now many sources of practical advice about communicating with disabled children with communication impairments. The list below is adapted from the one in Morris (ch 5, 2002).

Appendix: sources of practical advice

ACE Centre
This serves the south of England and Wales. Its mission statement includes the following key aim: 'To provide a child centred, multidisciplinary, independent assessment, advice and training service to the parents and carers of children with complex disabilities who require assisted/augmented communication aids in order to communicate and to learn.'

Address: The ACE Centre Advisory Trust,
92 Windmill Road, Headington, Oxford OX3 7DR.
Telephone: 01865 759800
Website: www.ace-centre.org.uk

ACE Centre North
Its website says 'ACE Centre North offers free information and advice on Assistive
Technology for people with physical/communication difficulties. This service is open to
all.' It serves the North of England.

Address: ACE Centre North, Hollinwood Business Centre,
Albert Street, Hollinwood
Oldham, OL8 3QL.
Tel: 0161 684 2333
Website: www.ace-north.org.uk

British Educational Communications and Technology Agency (Becta)
Their website states 'Becta leads the national drive to inspire and lead the effective and
innovative use of technology throughout learning. It's our ambition to create a more
exciting, rewarding and successful experience for learners of all ages and abilities
enabling them to achieve their potential. . . In line with Government policy and the
e-strategy, Becta is driving the development of a broader agenda in relation to inclusion
and special educational needs inside Becta and with partners.'

Address: Becta, Millburn Hill Road,
Science Part, Coventry CV4 7JJ.
Telephone: 024 7641 6994
Website: www.becta.org.uk

Communication Matters
'Communication Matters is the UK Chapter of the International Society for
Augmentative and Alternative Communication (ISAAC) which focuses on the needs
of people with complex communication needs who may benefit from AAC systems to
maximise their opportunities and enhance their life. Augmentative and alternative
communication (AAC) systems includes eye pointing, gesture, signing, using
symbol/word boards, and electronic speech devices. Communication Matters is also
a member of Communications Forum, the UK's national information resource for
people who have communication impairment, as well as their enablers and service
providers.'

Address: c/o The ACE Centre, 92 Windmill Road,
Headington, Oxford OX3 7DR.
Telephone: 0845 456 8211
Website: www.communicationmatters.org.uk

Foundation for Assistive Technology (FAST)
Its website states it is 'the primary source of information about developments in assistive technology (AT) in the UK. The database is freely available online to the public and currently includes information on over 800 research projects. . . The AT Forum is a coalition of organisations representing AT users and carers, professional bodies, service providers, policy makers and industry. Its aim is to work strategically with stakeholders to improve AT services and raise the profile of AT among policy-makers, commissioners and providers.'

Address: FAST, 12 City Forum,
250 City Road, London EC1V 8AF.
Telephone: 020 7253 3303
Website: www.fastuk.org

I CAN
'I CAN is the children's communication charity. We work to foster the development of speech, language and communication skills in all children with a special focus on those who find this hard: children with speech, language and communication needs.'

Address: I CAN, 8 Wakley Street,
London EC1V 7QE.
Telephone: 0845 225 4071
Website: www.ican.org.uk

Makaton
'Makaton is an internationally recognised communication programme used in more than 40 countries worldwide. Makaton can help if a child has difficulties with understanding and speaking. Through Makaton, the child is able to develop important communication skills. Makaton uses speech and gesture, facial expression, eye contact and body language.'

Address: The Makaton Charity, 31 Firwood Drive,
Camberley, Surrey GU15 3QD.
Telephone: 01276 61390
Website: www.makaton.org

Signalong Group
The Group is 'committed to empowering children and adults with impaired communication to understand and express their needs, choices and desires by providing vocabulary for life and learning. [It] strives to achieve this by developing and promoting augmentative communication (manual signs, symbols, picture resources). . .by teaching communication techniques to anyone living or working with people with impaired communication.'

Address: The Signalong Group, Stratford House,
Waterside Court, Rochester, Kent, ME2 4NZ.

Telephone: 0845 4508422
Website: www.signalong.org.uk

Triangle
This 'is an independant organisation that works with children and young people,
providing training and consultancy throughout the UK. . .Most of our work is around
children's rights, child protection, consultation, communication and inclusion. . .Much
of our work is with children who are disabled or have special educational needs and is
informed by a social model perspective on disability.'

Address: Unit E1, The Knoll Business Centre,
Old Shoreham Road, Hove, East Sussex BN3 7GS.
Telephone: 01273 413141
Website: www.triangle-services.co.uk

Chapter 10

Child Protection

Pat Cawson

Learning to think the unthinkable

The possibility that disabled children might be vulnerable to abuse or neglect reached the professional consciousness much later than happened with other children. Explanations for this may be in part because the structure of services often led to a separation between those for disabled children and their families and those focused on child protection, so that child protection specialists in all professions understood little about disability, while disability specialists were not familiar with child protection issues (National Working Group on Child Protection and Disability 2003). Some commentators have also suggested that practitioners and researchers are reluctant to think the unthinkable: disabled children occupy a social position that defines them as innocent and vulnerable and therefore bound to arouse protective and caring responses rather than abusive or uncaring responses. Sir William Utting, former Chief Social Services Inspector for England and Wales, wrote of the struggle he and his colleagues had with their own 'barriers of disbelief' when dealing with the aftermath of child abuse scandals in care services, particularly in accepting that members of the caring professions could abuse children:

> *Most difficult of all to accept was that disabled children could be victimized physically and become the targets of systematic sexual abuse. It was simply unthinkable that adults who had caring responsibilities could exploit and abuse children with physical, intellectual or sensory impairments. The evidence of inquiries, however, particularly into schools and other residential settings, demonstrated not only the reality of such abuse but also that it was almost impossible for disabled children to obtain redress through the criminal courts.*
> **(National Working Group on Child Protection and Disability 2003:7)**

The public inquiries into scandals in residential settings in the UK, and the earliest research, carried out predominately in the USA, showed how wrong the stereotypes were. There are definitional issues about disability as well as about maltreatment affecting prevalence studies, and there is still a dearth of reliable information internationally on the prevalence and incidence of the abuse of disabled children, compared with that available for children in the general population. Because severe childhood disability is rare, a general population sample is not the ideal method for assessing prevalence among the most severely disabled children, and studies have used a variety of different approaches to sampling. However, there is evidence from several countries that disabled children are more vulnerable to abuse than others, both in their families and when away from home (Westcott and Jones 1999). Pioneering research by Crosse et al (1993) and Sullivan and Knutson (1998) in the USA, using child protection agency and hospital based samples, showed much higher levels of abuse and neglect for disabled than for non-disabled children. Sullivan and Knutson's study using a school population of 40 000 children, established a 9% prevalence rate in the USA for non-disabled children and 31% for disabled children, with the highest levels for emotional abuse and neglect and the lowest for sexual abuse.

In the UK, a national study of the prevalence of child maltreatment, using retrospective self-report by a random probability sample of 2869 young people in the general population, also found that disabled young people were more likely to have experienced abuse and neglect (Cawson 2002). Young people had to use a laptop computer to take part in the study, excluding some of the most severely disabled, but 4% of respondents reported that they had a disability or long-term illness before the age of 16. In contrast to the USA results, the most marked difference was in sexual abuse, where 22% of disabled respondents experienced sexual abuse[1] by someone outside the family who was known to the child, compared with 15% of the sample as a whole. (Abusers were usually boyfriends, friends of the family, neighbours or fellow students, and very few respondents, disabled or non-disabled, reported abuse by professionals). In common with other self-report studies of sexual abuse, in the UK and elsewhere, two-thirds of respondents had told no one of the abuse at the time. This probably explains much of the difference between the UK findings and USA studies based on official records of abuse. Evidence on the abuse of more severely disabled children in the UK is available from Morris (1999), who established that although disabled children made up 2% of the child population in the areas she studied, they comprised 10% of the children on child protection registers.

Improving safeguards for disabled children
One consequence of opening up the care of disabled children to greater scrutiny has been a realisation of the poor quality of records concerning maltreatment and many other aspects of their care. Although local authorities are required to maintain registers of disabled children in order to identify their support needs, until recently the requirement was widely ignored. Where registers did exist they were incomplete

---

1   Defined as sexual acts occurring against the child's wishes or involving another person five or more years older, when the child was aged 12 or under.

(Department of Health 2001). Cooke (2000) surveyed social services UK wide, and found that although 51% of local authorities said that they recorded when a child on the child protection register was disabled, only 14% could give a figure for their own area. Recent government initiatives have been designed to improve information monitoring in order to give a good evidence base for services and to assess progress towards improved services. The Protection of Children Act 1999 and the Care Standards Act 2000 introduced new measures to strengthen safeguards for children by providing for the checking of criminal records of those working with children, and for national minimum standards for a range of social care and education services for children. Reports suggest that, although there has been improvement, there is still a long way to go in obtaining the information and resources needed for improvement of services for disabled children (*Quality Protects* (www.dcsf.gov.uk/qualityprotects) and Khan and Stuart 2000)

Research and practitioner experience in child protection services, however, has identified several ways in which disabled children are likely to be vulnerable to maltreatment. Particular concerns are as follows:

- Poor support to children and families, generally and where children are known to be at risk. Problems include:
    - failure by local education authorities to monitor placements when children are placed in special boarding schools (Abbott et al 2000, 2001),
    - failure by social services departments to support families of special school pupils when children return home for school holidays or when they leave school,
    - failure by social services to visit or give other support to disabled children Looked After or accommodated under the Children Act 1989 when placed in special boarding schools (Abbott et al 2000, 2001, Morris 1995, 1998) or in long-stay hospitals (Stalker et al 2003),
    - uncertainty by both social services and hospital staff about the legal status of children in long-stay hospital care (most of whom are severely disabled), resulting in some children effectively being abandoned in hospital with no one accepting parental responsibility (Stalker et al 2003).
- Lack of awareness of disability issues among social workers, health practitioners and police working in child protection services. Physical and behavioural indicators of abuse and neglect can be dismissed as resulting from the child's disability (for example as self-injury) rather than being recognized for what they are.
- Unfamiliarity of practitioners in relevant services with methods for communicating with children who have limited or no speech, and/or who primarily use non-verbal signing and symbol systems. Practitioners may be uncomfortable with non-verbal communication or reluctant to find and work with interpreters, thereby denying the child the opportunity to tell anyone about the abuse and neglect they are experiencing. The barrier to communication may be made more acute because some signing and symbol systems have limited vocabulary for describing abusive, especially sexual acts, although this is now being addressed by producers of most systems.

- Assumptions that children with communication or intellectual impairments will be unable to give evidence and that there is consequently no point in pursuing child protection enquiries or police investigations. This can deny children access to legal and other protection or redress and leave an abuser free to target other victims. (National Working Group on Child Protection and Disability 2003)

Safeguarding disabled children in residential settings

Disabled children are especially likely to spend part of their childhood living away from home, in respite foster care, children's homes, hospitals and hospices, and most of all in boarding schools. Again, there is a dearth of comprehensive and consistent information (Paul and Cawson 2002). The Office for Population Censuses and Surveys (OPCS) national survey of disabled children living at home and in communal establishments (comprising 3% of the child population) is now nearly 20 years old but is still the most recent available (Bone and Melzer 1989). The data showed that most disabled children in the UK had more than one disability, and that 20% had severe and multiple disabilities. The most severely disabled children were the most likely to enter care at a young age (Loughran et al 1992). The Department of Health has reported that 'there is a marked association between the number of disabilities a child has and the chances of being looked after in a residential setting' (Department of Health 2001). A government study attempted to estimate the numbers of disabled children boarding in special schools, looked after by local authorities and placed for prolonged periods in health care settings in 2002/3. The figures from different settings are difficult to compare, but suggest that between 8000 and 9000 disabled children are in residential placements at any one time (Department for Education and Skills (DfES) 2004a). The most vulnerable children are therefore most likely to be cared for away from home in residential settings, where they can be at risk for a variety of reasons. Children in residential settings with high physical dependency experience multiple carers and are likely to require intimate personal care. Children may be physically less able to resist abusers, and learning disabled children are more vulnerable to coercion and psychological pressure. Children in some boarding schools may have as many as 40 carers (Utting 1997). Residential settings may be physically isolated and many disabled children will be unable to access means of help, including helplines such as ChildLine and other direct access services. Parents may be out of contact or at such a distance that they are unable to see what is happening or communicate with the child. Physical and social isolation of some residential settings can lead to inward looking practice, and working unsocial hours makes it difficult for staff to have contact with other care settings or to undertake training. Management and staffing problems in residential settings can lead to recruitment of people who are not suited to the work, to poor staff support and training, and to staff working under pressure with poor resources (Support Force for Children's Residential Care 1995). Audits show that problems in recruitment and management are far from solved (National Care Standards Commission 2004).

As well as direct physical or sexual abuse, poor practice can become abusive if unchecked, and practices are accepted with disabled children that would be regarded as abusive with other children. The National Working Group on Child Protection and

Disability (2003) give examples of practice in the use of medication, in feeding children and in tying children into chairs, which would not be considered acceptable with non-disabled children. Morris gives a telling example of abusive bullying from a care home for young disabled people. A resident described the behaviour of a careworker:

> *'Sometimes' he said, 'I thought I was being stupid because he would make a joke out of it, and other people would think it was a joke, the things he said. The worst thing was not knowing when he would decide not to help me go to the toilet. He would say things like "oh you're always wanting a pee, there must be something wrong with you" or "have you been out drinking". They would think it was funny'.*

> *(Morris 1998)*

Although most of the attention in major scandals and public enquiries into institutions has focused on abuse by staff, there is some evidence from some residential settings that risk of harm from other residents may be greater (Barter et al 2004). Again, there is limited UK evidence specifically concerning disabled children, compared with that for non-disabled children, but a small study produced similar findings (Westcott 1993).

What is good safeguarding practice? Evidence from residential special schools

A study of practice in residential schools for children with severe and multiple disabilities explored staff experience and the issues that arose for practitioners in trying to ensure safe care for some of the most vulnerable children living in residential settings.[2] Schools were chosen to be broadly representative of the national picture, including schools of varying sizes, those from the maintained and independent sectors, and different parts of the country, but their participation in the project meant that they were committed to improving their own child protection practice. Some were part of larger organizations providing several schools, and others were small local charities. Some were exclusively for children with severe/multiple disabilities, and others admitted these children as part of a wider pupil group, on the basis of a specific disability. All took both boys and girls and all except one admitted primary and secondary age children, the remaining school being for secondary pupils. Some children were weekly or termly boarders, while others were in 52-week care, with their schools having dual registration as schools and children's homes. Full details of sampling and methods are given in the report on the research (Paul et al 2004). Eight schools took part in the main fieldwork. Three others helped with pilot work and by arranging for the researchers to talk to groups of children with verbal communication about what were their important issues for feeling safe and happy at school.

2 The fieldwork was carried out by the NSPCC Child protection Research Department from 1999–2002 and funded by the Community Fund (now the Big Lottery Fund).

Researchers spent a week in each school, joining in with school life from breakfast to bedtime, observing and talking to children and staff. Semi-structured tape recorded interviews were held with a selection of managers, staff, and governors or trustees, and researchers read and analysed relevant policy documents and procedure manuals. All participants were told that information given to the researchers would be confidential unless the researchers learned that a child was at serious risk, in which case action would be taken to protect the child, and a suitable management contact for this purpose was negotiated with each school.

Staff accounts of trying to mobilize community services when there were potential child protection concerns reflected the problems described above. Many pupils had difficult family situations and when children displayed evidence of problems arising on visits home or outside the school staff did not always get the back up they needed from local services or professionals in the child's home area. They encountered practitioners who understood little about severely learning disabled children, and services that were reluctant to support families when children were at home for the holidays. The same could happen if problems arose in school and help was sought from local child protection or health services. Potential indicators of abuse were often ascribed by professionals to the child's disability, and not regarded as they would have been with a non-disabled child.

> *On examination the doctor had not been concerned that there was accompanied bruising around his thighs and she assumed he had poked himself with a foreign object.*
>
> *(Head of Care)*

> *The boy displayed sexualized behaviour at a very early stage of development. He had no communication. We were deeply suspicious and concerned about the family dynamics. Initially the Child Protection team were in denial about the root of the sexual behaviour. Social services and the mental health team saw his behaviour as part of his autistic spectrum disorder.*
>
> *(Head of Care)*

At times complaints could be 'cooled out' or discouraged, especially if the child had little or no verbal communication, because it was assumed that no evidence could stand up to investigation.

> *There was an autistic boy who was putting dolls in positions that didn't leave much room for imagination . . . I went to see the Child Protection co-ordinator to relay what staff were observing and reporting. We were told that it probably wouldn't lead anywhere as you couldn't get a statement from the child.*
>
> *(Careworker)*

All the schools we visited raised the concern that communication and comprehension ability compromised the progress of child protection enquiries.

Occasionally, support was available to children from independent representation outside the school. Children looked after by local authorities in England and Wales have a right to independent visitors (Children Act 1989) if they have little or no contact with parents, though research suggests this provision is insufficiently used, especially for disabled children (Knight 1998, Winn Oakley and Masson 2000). Some voluntary organizations provide independent representative or advocate schemes, when an advocate will be attached to a particular school or children's home to work with all the children, and some local authorities employ children's rights officers whose role is to act as children's advocates if they are unhappy about something that has happened to them. Only one school in the study had a formal independent representation scheme attached to the school, and one maintained school was provided by a local education authority that had an advocate for all disabled children in the authority's schools.

Safe child protection systems
Good awareness of child protection issues was a prerequisite of safe practice, and the lead given by the head teachers and other senior managers was crucial. Most schools had a holistic approach to child protection, and stressed the importance of good communication with children:

> *I tell my staff that they have a shared responsibility to whistle-blow and I try and talk to them about the fact that child protection isn't just about burns and bruises but its about how we value, how we talk and how we care for the youngsters.*
>
> *(Head of Care)*

> *90% of our communication is not speech – it's body language and facial expression. And when you work with nonverbal students it becomes absolutely imperative. . .I noticed this morning with a student that he's not right – I don't know whether he's ill. He's nonverbal – so I noted it and recorded it on the shift report to say he's not happy, he's not right. Please keep a close eye.*
>
> *(Teacher)*

In some schools, however, the picture was less positive. Staff spoke of poor communication between staff or of not having access to information on child protection.

> *I expect we do have a designated child protection person but I couldn't tell you exactly who that was.*
>
> *(Careworker)*

There was a great dependence on good recording at all levels of school life because of the numbers of people involved in children's care and the children's often limited verbal communication. Most schools had a separate reporting procedure for child protection concerns, with specially designed forms, but some used incident forms or logs that could be used for many other purposes, and then it was not always possible to tell what if any action had followed the report. When dedicated report forms were available in each classroom and house unit, staff could make speedy records of worrying observations or incidents. If forms and logs were held only at a central point in the school, this made it harder to record issues at the time they cropped up, and engendered an attitude that child protection concerns were not matters of urgency.

> *I'd leave it to the key worker to follow this up and maybe a day later check that he had.*
>
> *(Teacher)*

Three elements stood out as characterizing schools which had the safest practice:

- a whistleblowing culture;
- no blame approaches;
- support for staff when allegations are made.

WHISTLEBLOWING

With a whistleblowing culture staff felt free to question and report behaviour by colleagues and seniors. This needs sensitive handling by management, openness about what will happen and a clear channel for who should receive and act on the reports.

> *We have had several people come and say they're not happy with what they have seen, which is spot on. . .what I always say to people as well is that they must be sure that either the head or myself are going to do something about it.*
>
> *(Head of Care)*

Researchers were told of and observed examples where whistleblowing had identified practice problems at an early stage. Where there was no such culture, or uncertainty about who to go to, or what would happen, staff were reluctant to challenge poor practice. In some schools, a rigid hierarchy and distant approach made it hard for staff to challenge long established or senior staff, and inexperienced staff could be persuaded that the poor practice they saw was 'normal' or necessary.

> *Sometimes schools have staff that have been there for a long time and it's all very archaic and there is this awful ranking where people are scared to stick their neck out.*
>
> *(Careworker)*

> *If somebody who has been in work for a long time and is probably a senior member of staff it is very difficult to expect a junior member of staff to complain about them.*
>
> *(Careworker)*

'NO BLAME' APPROACHES

A 'no blame' approach is clearly not appropriate in a situation where, for example, abuse by a predatory paedophile is discovered or suspected. However, problems that arise in residential services are frequently the result of staff uncertainty about good practice or to pressures on resources. Given the largely untrained workforce that currently typifies residential care, it is essential that issues can be taken up in a training and development context, in which staff can learn from mistakes, rather than be fearful of admitting them. With a no blame approach, reports could be dealt with sensitively, with help and guidance to staff who had made genuine mistakes or who did not realize their practice was problematic. Staff were enabled to ask for help if there was something they were finding it hard to cope with.

SUPPORT FOR STAFF AGAINST WHOM ALLEGATIONS ARE MADE

A lack of support to staff when allegations were made has been identified as a management problem in public enquiries and investigations of abuse (Barter 1998). In a close residential community, staff relationships and good teamwork are crucial to effective practice. Consequently, if staff see colleagues being treated unfairly or uncaringly by managers following mistakes or allegations, they are less likely to seek help with their own difficulties and are likely to be reluctant to 'grass up' their colleagues in future. Dealing with possible misconduct by staff can be a complex issue, especially if formal disciplinary or criminal procedures are instigated, and schools sometimes found that when external agencies became involved, the managers lost control of the process. Having someone assigned to liaise and support staff became very important to maintaining morale. One staff member described the difficulties experienced after an allegation.

> *I felt I was dealt with badly by the management and by Social Services because I was left to stew for 6 weeks not knowing what was going to happen. It wasn't until the first day back after the school holidays that I had a letter saying I was being called to a disciplinary hearing.*
>
> *(Staff member)*

Managing behaviour

The research found that two aspects of practice created specific child protection issues with these severely disabled children. These were: the management of children's sexuality, especially in relation to normal adolescent development and to children's need for demonstrative physical affection; and the response to challenging behaviour, including aggressive, sexualized or self-harming behaviour.

Affection and sexuality

Achieving a balance between ensuring children's safety, coping with their normal developmental needs for affection, and with developing adolescent sexuality, seemed to be the aspect of care that staff found most difficult, and to have the least support from school systems. This is a difficult aspect of childrearing for anyone charged with parental or other carer responsibilities, but for staff working with these severely disabled children it was especially testing. Anxiety about the risk of sexual abuse or about possible misconstructions of behaviour can lead to defensive practice which is really about protecting staff from allegations, rather than protecting children, and to rules that staff find hard to accept.

> *There is a policy about affection. . .The management team have said. . .any close contact should be minimal as it leaves us open to allegations. We don't*

keep physical attention to minimal, if these kids want affection they get it. They are only 9 and 10 – they are only little boys. . .we are like substitute parents.

(Careworker)

Practice and guidance on dealing with affectionate physical contact with children and with students' developing sexuality varied greatly between and within schools.

Schools had difficulty over deciding what display of physical affection should be allowed from or to students, especially as students often spent longer at school than at home and some children were in 52-week care. Some pupils were very young chronologically as well as intellectually impaired – all schools except one took primary and secondary pupils, and some had preschool programmes. Adolescents could be physically mature but developmentally much younger than their chronological age. Although sex education was one of the few areas where all schools had formal written policies, there was limited availability of helpful educational materials for such severely disabled children, especially when reliant on signing or symbol communication.

Physical affection was a particularly sensitive issue with adolescents, and in some schools, age-inappropriate behaviour was seen which made both students and staff potentially vulnerable.

You've probably seen me kissing P and I know I'm not supposed to. I am very touchy feely – that's my personality. I may be criticized for it and sometimes I know I've gone too far. I don't go up and kiss Y because I know he doesn't like close contact but P likes it – it focuses him and he really responds.

(Careworker)

Some schools had what was almost a complete prohibition on affectionate physical contact with pupils. Staff sometimes ignored their school's guidance because it seemed to them to defy common sense, or to deny children's need for affectionate touch. If the available guidance was seen as unrealistic and ignored, effectively there were no rules. This gave the wrong messages about acceptable sexual behaviour to intellectually and socially immature adolescents. Schools with best practice acknowledged children's need for affection and taught both staff and children acceptable ways to deal with it.

You have to consider their age. The difficulty is that staff see teenagers as kids but they are adults. You don't go round kissing people willy nilly. . .you don't have to repel them either – you could use a reassuring touch such as an arm around the shoulder. We teach our students appropriate hugs which mean affection.

(Teacher)

There is no simple right or wrong answer to this dilemma – no 'one size fits all' solution. It is important that any action is part of a planned response to the child, but one that does not stifle spontaneity. It is also very important that solutions are placed in a context of child development. Some of these children *were* very young, and most spent more of their time with care staff than with parents. Perhaps they shouldn't – but they do, and good care must acknowledge the reality of that.

Another problem area for staff was in dealing with overtly sexual behaviour by and between students. Lack of staff awareness and use of inappropriate intervention in some schools was a major concern. The researchers contrasted what they saw in some schools with the much more open approach to sexuality with learning disabled adults, and the greater availability of training and guidance for those working with adults. The schools often had great anxiety about sexual behaviour between pupils and were also anxious about whether attempts to teach pupils to express their sexuality in appropriate ways could be misinterpreted by observers and leave staff open to suspicion. There were occasions when the inability to deal with sexuality led to practice which could be seen as abusive. In one school, care staff used arm splints on a 17-year-old boy who was constantly trying to masturbate. When another staff member enquired the reason for this, they justified it by saying that 'the boy would otherwise get his hands inside the pad and soil everywhere'.

Public sexual behaviour was a common problem, but some schools were able to accept and address adolescent sexuality and develop strategies to help students deal with it.

> we've tended to, accept (masturbation), we have tried to clearly say to the child I understand that you want to, but you can only do this in your bedroom and now it is school time, we would schedule it into their timetable – the first thing on their schedule when they came home.
>
> *(Teacher)*

There were some schools where staff put a lot of thought into possible reasons for sexual behaviour which appeared damaging or obsessive, and looked for explanations and solutions, but others where the response was defensive practice. It seemed harder for staff to address open or destructive sexual behaviour than to address other challenging behaviour, where there was an impressive understanding of possible causes and triggers for behaviour and the messages that the behaviour could reflect.

Challenging behaviour

In giving safe responses to challenging behaviour the importance of communication issues cannot be overstressed, especially with children who lack speech. Staff were in general aware, versatile and focused on understanding what students were trying to tell them. It was important to record normality for the child, in order to identify when there was a problem.

> It's not unusual to be scratched, bitten or hair pulled. . .What we try and do is work out where the behaviour is coming from – It's not intended to hurt or upset you – it's because the child doesn't have a way of expressing their anger or frustration and it's our job to reduce that anger or frustration.
>
> *(Teacher)*

*If a child was being aggressive towards a particular staff member I would
wonder if they were trying to communicate they were upset or scared of them.
I know it's important not to jump to the possibility of abuse immediately but I
would consider abuse issues.*

(Careworker)

Most schools had detailed behaviour management plans for each student, which
travelled with the student from residential unit to classroom and sometimes to parents
during holidays. The schools that specialized in working with children who exhibited
high levels of challenging behaviour had the best practice in terms of behaviour
management. Training was given in behaviour management and physical intervention.
Worrying practice was sometimes found in schools where there were only a small
number of challenging children. In some schools there were concerns about the way
that challenging behaviour was managed by physical restraint, when staff had little or
no formal training in appropriate methods for the children they were dealing with. A
lack of formal training was found in schools where only a small number of children
required physical intervention

*The girl was face down at the time and we'd kept her there with one side of her
up against the skirting board so that she had one arm trapped. We had to sit it
out for 45 minutes.*

(Careworker)

In schools with good practice the researchers found:

● a group with specific responsibility for behaviour management – responsible for
formulating, implementing and monitoring plans, generally and for individual
students;

● the group had representatives from senior management, care and teaching staff;

● plans were clear and accessible and signed;

● plans were externally ratified by behaviour management professionals, the head,
parents and (in one school) the local authority;

● any changes made to plans were sanctioned by these professionals;

● systematic recording monitored challenging behaviour and physical intervention.

Effective plans identified and monitored likely triggers for aggressive or other problem
behaviour; gave detailed guidance on how to respond, had a good repertoire of
prevention and distraction techniques and emphasized that physical intervention must
only be used as a last resort. Staff were well prepared rather than having to react on the
hoof.

Working towards safer care
The commitment of the staff interviewed towards the children they were caring for
was impressive. Although some poor practice was found, this was the exception, and

continuous striving towards improved care was far more characteristic of the schools in this research. The findings carry a number of implications for the safeguarding of disabled children, in residential settings and elsewhere.

First comes the importance of 'hands on' management by senior staff. Best practice was found where the senior staff were available to support and encourage staff without taking over from them or undermining them. Poorer practice was found when seniors operated a 'nine to five' office based work pattern, and were rarely seen in the classrooms or house units. Senior involvement in monitoring child protection records and behaviour management with challenging children, and their modelling of good communications set the tone for the whole atmosphere of the school.

Second come questions of training. Most of the problem areas were amenable to good training, but managers and staff commented on the difficulty of finding external training suited to their needs. Little was available on specialist topics such as dealing with adolescent sexuality or challenging behaviour. Most schools had to rely on in-service training in the schools, creating the risk of encouraging inward looking practice. Schools that were part of larger specialist disability organizations fared best, but some schools were expected, by their managing agency or by their inspectors, to go through local training programmes which were geared to the needs of mainstream schools, and were largely irrelevant to the residential situation or the needs of severely disabled children. This was a problem when time and funding for training were scarce resources.

The shortage of specialist materials for educating children who have severe learning disabilities about their bodies and about sexual behaviour is a cause for concern, as is the equal dearth of practice information for professionals caring for them. Learning disabled children are exceptionally vulnerable to sexual exploitation and abuse and need more rather than less help than other children in coping with physical maturity. This must impact on children living in the community as well as those away from home. Learning disabled children are over represented in services for young sexual abusers and practitioners in these services have also described the limitations of existing resources to work with them (Hackett et al 2003). It seems likely that for some children, vulnerability to sexual abuse and exhibiting inappropriate sexual behaviour are two sides of the same coin, contributed to by poor preparation on sexuality and acceptable sexual behaviour.

The finding on challenging behaviour also raise questions about placement choice and the availability of suitable specialist care for the most challenging children within a reasonable distance of a child's home. In most services where there are just a few hundred children nationally with complex needs, rare medical conditions or exceptional behaviour we expect to find a national approach, if not to service provision at least to networking, referral and training. With children who have the most severe disabilities and challenging behaviour, however, there is no national overview of facilities, and only recently have there been attempts to establish any national and comprehensive data on residential school resources. There is clearly a need for a national perspective on the care, protection and educational needs of these children, rather than having all development left to local services that may have only one or two children at any one time with such extreme and complex needs.

Finally, good support from outside the residential setting is essential if children are to be safe and defensive practice avoided. On site managers and staff need the confidence that external management agencies, their inspection bodies and local services will take the children's need for protection seriously. They also need back up from external professionals who will understand children's developmental needs and behaviour, and support staff in making reasonable professional decisions, rather than expecting a risk-free and sterile environment for the sake of protecting the staff or management from any possible criticism or allegation. Children need the possibility of communication with someone from outside the residential setting if they are unable to contact parents or other sources of help, and feel unable to confide in staff. Since the research was carried out the Commission for Social Care Inspection has established a children's rights director whose role includes acting on behalf of children in residential homes or schools who contact him, and this service is being used regularly by children with access to telephones and email. However, few children in the present study would have been able to access this service directly. Children with severe disabilities and limited communication can only use independent visitors or advocates as a protection from abuse or poor practice if the service is delivered directly to them, and this is a service that they should be able to expect from all local authorities.

Chapter 11

Children with Special Health Care Needs in Foster Care in the United States

Moira Szilagyi

Introduction

The United States (USA), like the United Kingdom (UK), has children for whom out-of-home care is deemed essential for issues of safety or health. Out-of-home care in both countries is intended to be a time of healing for children and families and a window of opportunity during which families can acquire services they need to successfully reunite with their children. The governments of both countries have responded in recent years to the growing body of evidence about what children need to thrive, passing legislation intended to provide for the needs of children in out-of-home care, protect them and foster permanency for them. However, in both countries, much remains to be done, especially on behalf of the subset of children with severe disabilities and their families. This vulnerable population of children tends to remain in the care system longer, and many grow up in public care as their families fade out of their lives. While there are many similarities among how our two countries care for disabled children and their families, there are also some differences, and it is the latter this chapter focuses on.

In the USA, children in out-of-home care are predominantly the children of the poor and disenfranchised. They are children who have endured abuse and/or neglect, and for whom out-of-home care is intended to be a temporary respite. As a group, children entering out-of-home care, have very high rates of chronic medical illness, mental health issues, developmental delays and educational disabilities. They have not received the normal, predictable nurturance deemed essential for optimal development and well-being. Their parents have high rates of mental illness, substance addiction, criminal involvement, and unemployment.

Out-of-home care for children in the USA is referred to as foster care, regardless of how children or adolescents arrive there or where they live.

- The foster care population in the USA is about 10 times that of the UK, numbering just over 510 000 children in foster care daily, over 800 000 per year. This reflects a somewhat higher per capita rate of removal than the UK.
- Unlike the UK, the rate of *voluntary* placement of children in foster care by families is quite low, ranging around 1% (versus 30%). The small number of children and adolescents placed voluntarily in the USA are those with complex mental or physical health needs, whose parents lack the capacity or resources to care for them.
- Overall, in the USA, 70% of children in foster care are placed *involuntarily* for reasons of child abuse and neglect.
- Almost all the remainder are adolescents placed *involuntarily* for reasons of juvenile delinquency or 'person in need of supervision'.
- Thus, the population of children in out-of-home care in the USA is essentially there because of *involuntary* court-ordered placement.

The goals of foster care are to ensure the safety and health of children while seeking timely permanency for them. In the USA, about 60% of children return to their family of origin, 20% are eventually adopted, and 18% age out of foster care. There are about 120 000 children in foster care awaiting adoption, and about half of those have an identified adoptive parent, who is, almost always, their foster parent. Others are awaiting adoption by a relative. About 60 000 children awaiting adoption are mostly older minority children, members of large sibling groups, and those with severe developmental disabilities and/or behavioural issues. A very small percentage of this group are children with medically complex conditions who are technology-dependent.

In the USA, there is, of course, a subset of children and adolescents in foster care whose health issues are so significant as to place them in that unique category, called for the purposes of this book, disabled children. As in the UK, the number of children with severe developmental, behavioural and/or emotional conditions dwarfs those with complex physical health issues, sometimes also referred to as multiply-disabling conditions. The overall health status of the 510 000 children and adolescents in foster care in the USA is so poor that the American Academy of Pediatrics (AAP) now recognizes the entire foster care population as a population of 'children with special health care needs' (www.aap.org/healthtopics/fostercare.cfm). Given the high prevalence of chronic medical (35–60%), mental health (60–80% of children over age 4 years), developmental (60% of children under age 5 years), educational (45% of children 6–11 years) and dental (30–40%) health conditions, this designation is well-warranted, although it has yet to be translated into coherent policy or result in any re-allocation of health resources. The percentage of children with multiply-disabling conditions in foster care is actually not known, as the criteria qualifying a child for this designation are somewhat unclear and child welfare does not currently keep statistics on health conditions. Estimates range from 3% to 11% of the population, depending on how one defines such disabilities.

Finding appropriate foster care placements for children with severe health issues is challenging because of the lack of 'therapeutic' foster homes. Foster parents willing to take medically, developmentally or behaviourally complex children often receive minimal training or additional support beyond an enhanced foster care board rate. As in the UK, children with significant disabilities have longer lengths of stay in foster care, since they are less likely to return to their family of origin or to be adopted. In particular, foster care tends to accumulate children with complex mental health and developmental conditions, especially if they also are of minority ethnicity or older age. Major barriers to achieving permanency include a shortage of families willing to adopt children with complex conditions, the loss of access to some resources once a child is adopted, and a lack of respite services. It is not uncommon in the USA for the dually-diagnosed, those with mental retardation and severe behaviour issues, to grow up in foster care and end up, as adults, in the guardianship of the state. Children with complex medical issues fare far better in achieving permanency than children with complex developmental and behavioural issues, unless their health conditions are so severe as to pose an undue financial burden on an adoptive family.

In the USA, children in foster care with significant behavioural and developmental disabilities are also apt to have more foster home placements than other healthier children. Unlike the UK, where many children with complex disabilities reside in boarding schools, almost all such children in foster care in America reside with foster families, reflecting the dramatic decline in residential placements for disabled children generally in the USA over the last 40 to 50 years. In the USA, the focus is on keeping children with their families, or, for those in foster care, in a family-based setting. This practice is now supported by a large body of evidence that an appropriate family setting best meets children's needs for nurturance, a sense of belonging, and attachment to at least one primary caregiver. Children with complex medical conditions tend to have more stable foster home placements than children with severe behavioural and developmental issues. The largest challenge remains the shortage of foster parents with appropriate skills to care for a severely disabled child, regardless of the type of disability. Children in the general population with extreme developmental delay and behavioural issues may be cared for in small group home facilities, if they are unable to be cared for safely in a family setting, but waiting lists are long and payment is prohibitive if insurance does not cover it. These children remain in the legal guardianship of their families and there is no involvement of the government except to regulate the facility. About 18% of children in foster care are in residential placement or group home care, but almost all are adolescents with significant mental health and behavioural issues.

As in the UK, children in foster care with severe disabilities of any type are actually less likely to maintain contact with their birth families over time. Birth parents may experience guilt over placing their child in foster care, or feelings of inadequacy when a foster parent appears better able to meet their child's needs or manage their behaviour. The continued engagement of the birth parents in such situations over time requires compassionate and highly skilled caseworkers and foster parents.

Permanency became the predominant goal of foster care in the USA with passage of the Adoption and Safe Families Act of 1997 (ASFA), and the foster care agency is expected to step in to terminate parental rights if the birth parent(s) or extended family are unable to resume the care of the child in a reasonable amount of time. Federal law dictates that if a child has been in foster care for 15 of the previous 22 months, the state must begin proceedings to terminate parental rights. The state can opt out of this requirement if the parent is making significant efforts toward reunification. 'Kinship care' by relatives who are not certified foster parents has become an increasingly common placement option in the last decade, in an effort to prevent foster care placement and promote permanency. In some states, kinship providers are reimbursed but not regulated as foster parents are. In others, they are neither reimbursed nor regulated. Kinship providers who become certified foster parents are referred to as 'relative resource' placements and now account for about 30% of all foster care placements in some states. Overall, kinship care providers are older, poorer and have less access to services for themselves and children in their care. However, studies show that children in kinship care tend to have a more stable placement. Approximately four times as many children are in unregulated kinship care as in foster care, and, in general, they have the same health needs and conditions as children in foster care. There is no data available on how children with severe disabilities of any type fare in kinship care settings.

As in the UK, children with disabilities are more liable to be abused or neglected, and tend to enter foster care for all the usual reasons of child abuse and neglect. A small percentage of multiply disabled children, especially those who are technology-dependent, are voluntarily placed by parents overwhelmed by their child's care needs, limited resources, and a lack of respite services. However a child enters care, the risk of abuse and/or neglect in a foster home or a school setting is higher for a child with significant disabilities. Professionals must always be aware of this issue and health providers, according to AAP standards, should screen for abuse and neglect at every health encounter with a child in foster care.

Virtually all children entering foster care suffer great emotional trauma at the time of removal from their families. Even if removal is involuntary, most children beyond infancy experience feelings of rejection and loss. These feelings may be compounded by fear and anxiety about their parents and siblings and how they are faring, but also by guilt, anger and a sense of alienation. The trauma of ongoing separation and the uncertainty about their future and that of their family add to the emotional burden carried by children. Sometimes, the only child placed in foster care by an overwhelmed family is the special needs child. For children with disabilities, there is the dual stigma of being both a foster child and disabled, and being somehow less worthy and less lovable.

Evaluations and services

The resources available to families vary from state to state, and sometimes among localities within a state. More rural areas often lack certain services almost completely, and the demand in large urban areas may well exceed supply. While every child with a disability is supposed to have access to a case manager, the parent is often the one who assumes the burden of coordinating and managing a complex array of services, medical equipment procurement, evaluations, medications, in addition to providing most or all of the daily care.

Children under age 36 months with developmental disabilities or risk factors for future disability can receive a developmental evaluation through the nationally mandated *Early Intervention Program*. Children who qualify for services can then receive home-based or center-based services at government expense. For preschool and school-aged children, evaluations are conducted through, and at the expense of, the child's home school district special education programme. A child who has identified needs and meets certain criteria for eligibility has an *Individual Educational Plan* (IEP) and indicated services are provided by the school district. Children with developmental or educational conditions may also be referred to developmental pediatricians for diagnostic purposes, but access is challenging since most such professionals are found only at university medical centers.

Placement of a child in out-of-home care to access needed health services is a significant issue on both sides of the Atlantic. While complex physical disabilities are a common reason for placement in the UK, placement of a child in foster care to access adequate mental health services is the much larger issue in the USA. Older children with extreme mental health needs are sometimes placed to access services not covered by their family's health insurance. Mental health coverage by commercial (private) health insurance is sub-optimal, as there are limits on the duration and types of services and most have requirements for large co-payments at the time of use. Thus, in many states, families find themselves forced to place their troubled child or adolescent in foster care, often compounding the emotional issues of the adolescent and the family, to access appropriate outpatient or residential mental health services. The latter, if not covered by insurance, may cost $80 000–150 000 annually, an amount that is essentially unaffordable. Within a month of placement in foster care, almost every child becomes eligible for public health insurance, known as Medicaid in the USA, and the burden of cost is then assumed by the public sector

Barriers to accessing health care

For children in foster care, there are multiple barriers to accessing appropriate health and mental health evaluations and services, beginning with obtaining appropriate consent. In the USA, the commissioner of social services in each local district is *in loco parentis* for children placed in foster care involuntarily, and may sign consents for health care after attempts to include the legal guardian have been exhausted. However, the commissioner may not sign consent for either Early Intervention or special education evaluations or services. These particular consents must be signed by the child's legal guardian or educational surrogate. Children who change foster homes or move out of foster care may move out of the service area, and consent may not follow. While the IEP is supposed to follow the child, there can be delays in re-starting services in a new school district when home changes occur.

Other barriers to obtaining appropriate evaluations and services include the fact that many health practitioners do not accept Medicaid reimbursement because of under-reimbursement. Children in foster care are highly mobile, moving in and out of foster care, or among foster care placements, and care with a particular health practitioner may be interrupted when transitions occur. The dearth of historical health information, family health histories, and the lack of familiarity with the child by the current caregiver often mean that children do not receive all the services they need. Most paediatricians and family medicine doctors do not conduct a comprehensive health assessment when children enter foster care because they are unfamiliar with health care standards for this population or not aware of the high risk indicators in the child's past.

The foster care medical home concept

In the USA, there are a few centers of excellence, attempting to ensure that each child in foster care has a 'medical home' in their community. A 'medical home' is a primary care paediatric office that strives to meet certain goals designated by the AAP as essential. Medical homes are paediatric practices that are accessible, offer the family and child continuity of care that is compassionate, family-centered, child-focused, comprehensive, culturally competent, of high quality, and well-coordinated. In addition, foster care medical homes are paediatric practices serving children in foster care and are expected to have some expertise in child abuse and neglect and foster care, and the impact of both on the lives and well-being of children and families. These specialized foster care medical homes are also expected to communicate effectively across systems with child welfare, the judiciary, and mental health, in particular, about the child's health needs and how those needs should be met. The foster care medical home ideally serves multiple roles on behalf of children in foster care: health care provider, health educator, health care coordinator and health care advocate.

Health care coordination

The national health system of the UK, at least in theory, offers a distinct advantage to Looked After children in that each child appears to have access to a primary health care practitioner. This concept is in its infancy in the USA, where there is no systematic way in which children in foster care access health care, or even identify a primary health care provider. Some children remain with their primary care practitioner after entry to foster care, some change practitioners every time they experience a change in foster care placement, and some access health care on a crisis-oriented basis from a myriad of resources, most often from the emergency department. Occasionally, a foster care agency has a health practitioner who does 'intake evaluations'. Overall, health care for children in foster care is fragmented, lacks coordination, is not designed to identify or manage their health needs, and is not integrated with the child welfare system.

The coordination of health services for children in foster care is fundamental to ensuring that their multiple health issues are identified and addressed. In the USA, this task most often falls on the shoulders of the foster parent or caseworker, neither of whom is equipped to deal with accessing the array of services the child needs in America's complex and disjointed health care system. The single point of entry to health care should be the child's primary care physician, who is ideally a paediatrician. A special needs child should also have a health care coordinator available to them through their primary care practitioner, the local department of public health, social services or one of the developmental agencies providing services. However, in practice, it is the foster parent or caseworker who assumes this pivotal role for most children.

Health care management for children in foster care is a responsibility of the local child welfare agency but should be conducted by health professionals. In a few localities, foster care medical homes (centralized primary care paediatric offices described previously) provide all the primary health care and health care coordination for children while they are in foster care. Such foster care medical homes are paediatric offices that may be based in public health departments, university hospital clinics, or foster care agencies. They serve as a central repository for health care and health information that child welfare then has ready access to. This promotes the integration of health planning into the permanency plan for the individual child.

In some communities, foster care agencies address the health needs of children by conducting multidisciplinary intake evaluations to identify the spectrum of a child's health needs, and then allowing the foster parent to utilize their usual source of primary health care for children in their family. Unfortunately, most do not then subsequently track children to ensure that any identified health needs are met. At least three states have computerized health tracking systems for children in foster care and encourage health practitioners to communicate health information by providing standardized forms or access to a web-based health passport. Other localities rely on public health nurses to serve as health care coordinators, much like the clinical nurse specialist model in Caerphilly, Wales (see Chapter 4). However, overall, in the USA, child welfare and foster care agencies do not address the issues of health access, quality of care, coordination of health services, and health information sharing in any systematic manner, and the examples cited herein are isolated rather than routine.

Recommendations

Over the last 15 years, recommendations based on experience, research and best practice have been set forth by multiple professional organizations on improving health outcomes for children in foster care. In brief, those recommendations suggest the adoption of health care standards as outlined by the American Academy of Pediatrics (2005), and include:

- every child in foster care should have a medical home;
- every child in foster care should have a comprehensive medical evaluation shortly after entering foster care, ideally in their medical home;
- every child in foster care should receive preventive health care services on an enhanced schedule recommended by the AAP: that is, monthly to age 6 months, every 3 months until age 2 years, and then every 6 months;

- every child in foster care should have an evaluation by a specialized mental health professional at entry to care and at periodic intervals thereafter;
- every child in foster care should have an evaluation by a developmental/educational professional at entry to care and at periodic intervals thereafter;
- every child in foster care should have a health professional whose responsibility it is to coordinate the child's health care and collaborate closely with the foster care agency to ensure the child's needs are addressed and that health information is integrated into the permanency planning for the child.

Conclusions

In an ideal world, families would have access to the array of high-quality services they need to maintain their children with disabilities in their families. For children who need to be placed in out-of-home care, foster care done right should indeed buffer the impact of multiple chronic adverse childhood experiences and be, at the least, a window of opportunity for optimizing their health and well-being. Children living with disabilities residing away from family for whatever reason should not be defined by their disability, although the needs emanating from that disability should be met. Optimizing the health outcomes of disabled children in foster care should help child welfare meet its goals, including:

- providing each child with care in a family setting that is stable over time;
- maintaining contact between the child and the family of origin where desirable;
- offering each child a voice in the system entrusted with their care and well-being;
- achieving the ultimate goal of permanency in a 'forever family'; and
- fostering the growth of a healthy, resilient individual.

References

Abbott D, Morris J, Ward L. (2000) *Disabled Children and Residential Schools: A Survey of Local Authority Policy and Practice.* Bristol: Norah Fry Research Centre, University of Bristol.

Abbott D, Morris J, Ward L. (2001) *The Best Place to be?* York: Joseph Rowntree Foundation.

Abbott D, Townsley R, Watson D. (2005) Multiagency working in services for disabled children: what impact does it have on professionals? *Health Soc Care Community* **13**: 155–163.

Ainsworth M, Blehar M, Waters E, Wall S. (1978) *Patterns with Attachment: A Psychological Study of a Strange Situation.* Hillsdale, NJ: Lawrence, Elbaum.

Albers E, Riksen-Walraven M, Sweep F, de Weerth C. (2008) Maternal behavior predicts infant cortisol recovery from a mild everyday stressor. *J Child Psychol Psychiatry* **49**: 97–103.

Allen RE, Oliver JM. (1982) The effects of child maltreatment on language development. *Child Abuse Neglect* **6**: 299–305.

Ames J. (1996) Fostering children and young people with learning disabilities: the perspectives of birth children and carers. *Adoption and Fostering* **20**: 36–41.

American Academy of Pediatrics District II, Task Force on Health Care for Children in Foster Care and District II Committee on Early Childhood, Adoption and Dependent Care. (2005) Fostering Health: Health Care for Children and Adolescents in Foster Care. Elk Grove IL: AAP. (www.aap.org)

Ayoub C, Rappolt-Schlichtmann G. (2007) Child maltreatment and the development of alternative pathways in biology and behaviour. In: Coch D, Dawson, G, Fischer K, editors. *Human Behaviour, Learning and the Developing Brain. Atypical Development.* New York: Guildford Press. pp 305–325.

Bamford F, Wolkind SN. (1988) *The Physical and Mental Health Needs of Children in Care. Research Needs.* London: Economic and Research Council.

Baker BL, Blacher J. (2002) For better or worse? Impact of residential placement on families. *Ment Retard* **40**: 1–13.

Baker BL, Blacher J, Pfeiffer S. (1993) Family involvement in residential treatment of children with psychiatric disorder and mental retardation. *Hosp Community Psychiatry* **44**: 561–566.

Barter C. (1998) *Investigating Institutional Abuse.* London: NSPCC.

Barter C, Renold E, Berridge D, Cawson P. (2004) *Peer Violence in Children's Residential Homes.* Basingstoke: Palgrave.

Berney TP. (2000) Psychiatric Services. In: Gillberg C, O'Brien G, editors. *Developmental Disability and Behaviour.* Clinics in Developmental Medicine, Volume 149. London: Mac Keith Press. pp 159–170.

Besag VE. (1989) *Bullies and Victims in Schools: A Guide to Understanding and Management.* Milton Keynes: Open University Press.

Bone M, Meltzer H. (1989) *OPCS Survey of Disability in Great Britain Report 3: The Prevalence of Disability among Children.* London: HMSO.

Borthwick-Duffy SA, Widaman KP, Little TD, Eyman RK. (1992) Foster family care for persons with mental retardation. *Monogr Am Assoc Ment Retard* **17**: 154–156.

Bowlby J. (1969) *Attachment.* London: The Howarth Press.

Bremner J, Southwick S, Johnson D, Yehuda R, Charney D. (1993) Childhood psychical abuse and combat-related post traumatic stress disorder in Vietnam veterans. *Am J Psychiatry* **150**: 235–239.

British Association for Adoption and Fostering. (2007) *Summary Statistics on Children in Care and Children Adopted from Care, and Searching for Birth Relatives in England.* London: BAAF. (www.baaf.org.uk/info/stats/england.shtml)

Bundkle A. (2001)Health of teenagers in residential care: comparison of data held by care staff with data in community child health records. *Arch Dis Child* **84**: 10–14.

Butler I, Payne H. (1997) The health of children looked after by the local authority. *Adoption and Fostering* **21**: 28–35.

Butler I, Roberts G. (1997) *Social Work with Children and Families.* London: Jessica Kinsley Publishers.

Care Standards Act 2000. London: The Stationery Office. (www.opsi.gov.uk/acts/acts2000/ukpga_20000014_en_1.htm)

Carlile A. (2002) *Too Serious a Thing – A report on the Safeguards for Children Cared for and treated by the NHS in Wales – The Carlile Review.* Cardiff: Welsh Assembly Government.

Carlson V, Cicchetti D, Barnatt D, Braunwald K. (1989) Disorganised/disoriented attachment relationships in maltreated infants. *Dev Psych* **25**: 525–531.

Cawson P. (2002) *Child Maltreatment in the Family.* London: NSPCC.

Children Act 1989. London: The Stationery Office. (http://www.opsi.gov.uk/acts/acts1989/ukpga_1989 0041_en_1.)

Children Act 2004. London: The Stationery Office. (http://www.opsi.gov.uk/acts/acts2004/ukpga_2004 0031_en_1)

Children's Commissioner for Wales. (2004) *The Children's Commissioner for Wales Annual Report 2003–4.* Cardiff: Welsh Assembly Government.

Cooke P. (2000) *Final Report on Disabled Children and Abuse.* Nottingham: The Ann Craft Trust.

Corlyon J, McGuire C. (1997) *Young Parents in Public Care: Pregnancy and Parenthood among Young People Looked After by Local Authorities.* London: National Children's Bureau.

Council for Disabled Children. (1999) *Quality Protects: First Analysis of Management Action Plans with Reference to Disabled Children and Families.* London: DH.

Cousins J. (2006) *Every Child is Special: Placing Disabled Children for Permanence.* London: BAAF.

Cousins J. (2008) *Ten Top Tips for Finding Families for Children.* London: BAAF.

Cowen PS, Reed DA. (2002) Effects of respite care for children with developmental disabilities: evaluation of an intervention for at risk families. *Public Health Nurs* **19**: 272–283.

Crosse S, Kaye E, Ratnofsky A. (1993) *A Report on the Maltreatment of Children with Disabilities.* Washington, DC: National Centre on Child Abuse and Neglect.

de Bildt A, Serra M, Luteijn E, Kraijer D, Sytema S, Minderaa R. (2005) Social skills in children with intellectual disabilities with and without autism. *J Intellect Disabil Res* **49**: 317–328.

Department for Children, Schools and Families. (2008) *Children Looked After in England (including adoptions and care leavers) Year Ending 31 March 2008.* London: DCSF. (www.dcsf.gov.uk/rsgateway/DB/SFR/s000810/index.shtml)

Department for Education and Employment. (1999a) *Social Exclusion: Pupil Support. Circular 10/99.* London: DfEE.

References

Department for Education and Employment. (1999b) *Social Exclusion: Pupil Support, Trauancy and School Exclusion. Circular 11/99.* London: DfEE.

Department for Education and Skills. (2001) *The Special Educational Needs Code of Practice.* London: DfES.

Department for Education and Skills. (2003) *Every Child Matters.* London: DfES.

Department for Education and Skills. (2004a) *Disabled Children in Residential Placements.* London: The Stationery Office. (www.teachernet.gov.uk/docbank/index.cfm?id=6462)

Department for Education and Skills. (2004b) *Every Child Matters: Change for Children.* London: DfES.

Department for Education and Skills. (2004c) *Every Child Matters: Next Steps.* London: DfES.

Department for Education and Skills. (2004d) *Every Child Matters: Change for Children in Schools.* London, DfES.

Department for Education and Skills. (2004e) *Removing Barriers to Achievement: The Government's Strategy for SEN.* London: DfES.

Department for Education and Skills/Department of Health. (2000) *Education of Young People in Public Care.* London: DH.

Department for Education and Skills and the Department of Health. (2002) *Guidance on the Use of Restrictive Physical Interventions for Staff Working with Children and Adults who Display Extreme Behaviour in Association with Learning Disability and/or Autistic Spectrum Disorders.* London: Office of Public Sector Information.

Department for Education and Skills/National Statistics. (2004) *Statistics of Education: Outcome Indicators for Looked After Children: Twelve months to 30 September 2003.* England. London: The Stationery Office.

Department for Education and Skills/National Statistics. (2005) *Statistics of Education: Children Looked After in England 2003–2004.* National Statistics Bulletin, Issue no 01/05, January 2005. London: The Stationery Office. (http://www.dcsf.gov.uk/rsgateway/DB/SBU/b000552/CLAbulletin2003–04final.pdf)

Department of Health. (1991a) *Patterns and Outcomes in Child Placement: Messages from Current Research and their Implications.* London: HMSO.

Department of Health. (1991b) *The Children Act 1989 Guidance and Regulations, Volume 6, Children with Disabilities.* London: HMSO.

Department of Health. (1991c) *The Children Act 1989 Guidance and Regulations, Vol. 3, Family Placements.* London: HMSO. Section 9.36, p 94.

Department of Health. (1998) *Disabled Children: Directions for their Future Care.* London: HMSO.

Department of Health (1999) *Promoting the Health of Looked After Children: A Guide to Healthcare Planning, Assessment and Monitoring. A Consultation Document.* London: DH.

Department of Health. (2000) *Guidance to the Framework for the Assessment of Children in Need and their Families.* London: The Stationery Office.

Department of Health. (2001) *The Children Act Report.* London: DH. Ch 6, pp 32–34. (http://www.dh.gov.uk/en/Publicationsandstatistics/Publications/PublicationsLegislation/DH_4007485)

Department of Health. (2002a) *Promoting the Health of Looked After Children.* London: DH.

Department of Health. (2002b) *Residential Special Schools: National Minimum Standards. Inspection Regulations.* London: DH.

Department of Health. (2003) *Making Change Happen. The Government's First Annual Report on Learning Disability.* London: The Stationery Office.

Department of Health. (2004a) *National Service Framework for Children, Young People and Maternity.* London: The Stationary Office. (http://www.dh.gov.uk/en/Healthcare/NationalServiceFrameworks/Children/DH_4089111)

Department of Health. (2004b) *Key Issues for Primary Care. National Service Framework for Children and Young People and Maternity Services.* London: DH.

Department of Health. (2004c) *Disabled Children and Young People and Those with Complex Health Needs. National Service Framework for Children and Young People and Maternity Services.* London: DH.

Dimigen G, De Priore C, Butler S, Evans S, Ferguson L, Swan M. (1999) Psychiatric disorder among children at time of entering local authority care: questionnaire survey. *BMJ* **319**: 675.

Disabled Persons Act 1986. London: The Stationery Office.

Education Reform Act 1988. London: The Stationery Office.

England and Wales High Court (Family Division) Decisions. (2004) EWHC 2247 (Fam) FD04CO1788 between Portsmouth NHS Trust and Derek Wyatt and Charlotte Wyatt by her Guardian and Southampton NHS Trust.

Erickson MF, Egeland B. (1996) Child Neglect. In: Briere J, Berliner L, Bulkley JA, Jenny C, Reid T, editors. *The APSAC Handbook on Child Maltreatment.* Thousand Oaks, Ca: Sage Publications. pp 4–20.

Fleming P, Bamford DR, McCaughley N. (2005) An exploration of the health and social wellbeing needs of looked after young people- a multi-method approach. *J Interprof Care* **9**: 35–39.

Flynn R. (2002) *Short Breaks: Providing Better Access and More Choice for Black Disabled Children and their Parents.* Bristol: The Policy Press.

George RM, VanVoorhis J, Grant S, Casey K, Robinson M. (1992) Special education experience of foster children: an empirical study. *Child Welfare* **71**: 419–437.

Gero V, Sloper P, Barton K. (2004) *Key Worker Services for Disabled Children is Patchy. Research Findings.* York: Social Policy Research Unit, University of York.

Glaser D. (2000) Child abuse and neglect and the brain – a review. *J of Child Psychol Psychiatry* **41**: 97–116.

Goffman E. (1990) *Asylums: Essays on the Social Situation of Mental Patients and Other Inmates.* New York: Doubleday.

Goodman R, Scott S. (1999) Comparing the strengths and difficulties questionnaire and the child behaviour checklist. Is small beautiful? *J Abnorm Child Psychol* **27**: 17–24.

Gordon D, Parker R, Longhran F, Heslop P. (2000) *Disabled Children in Britain: A Re-analysis of the OPCS Disability Surveys.* London: The Stationery Office.

Gould J, Payne H. (2004) Health Needs of children in prison. *Arch Dis Child* **89**: 549–550.

Govindshenoy M, Spencer N. (2007) Abuse of the disabled child: a systemic review of population-based studies. *Child Care Health Dev* **33**: 552–558.

Green SE. (2004) The impact of stigma on maternal attitudes toward placement of children with disabilities in residential care facilities. *Soc Sci Med* **59**: 799–812.

Gunnar M. (2007) Stress effects on the developing brain. In: Romer D, Walker E, editors. *Adolescent Psychopathology and the Developing Brain.* Oxford: Oxford University Press. pp 133–215.

Hackett S, Masson H and Phillips S. (2003) *Mapping and Exploring Services for Young People who have Sexually Abused Others: Final Report.* Durham: University of Durham and University of Huddersfield.

Hall DMB, Elliman D. (2003) *Health for all Children*, 4th edn. Oxford: Oxford University Press.<Ch 3 AQ5>

Harris J, Allen D, Cornick M, Jefferson A, Mills R. (1996) *Physical Interventions: A Policy Framework.* Kidderminster: British Institute of Learning Disabilities.

Heath F, Smith R. (2004) *People Not Budgets.* London: The Centre for Policy Studies.

Hill CM, Mather M, Goddard J. (2003) Cross sectional survey of meningococcal C immunisation in children looked after by local authorities and those living at home. *BMJ* **326**: 364–365

Hill CM, Watkins J. (2003) Statutory health assessments for looked after children: what do they achieve? *Child Care Health Dev* **29**: 3–13.

Howell S. (2001) *The Health of Looked After Children, Highlight, 184.* London: National Children's Bureau.

Huang ZJ, Kogan MD, Yu SM, Strickland B. (2005) Delayed or forgone care among children with special health needs: and analysis of the 2001 National Survey of children with special health care needs. *Ambul Pediatr* **5**: 60–67.

Ivaldi G. (2000) *Surveying Adoption.* London: BAAF.

References

Jacobson JW. (1993) Public policy and the punishment of the powerless. Special issue: aversives. *Child and Adolescent Mental Health Care* **3**: 7–18.

Johnson CP, Kastner TA, American Academy of Pediatrics Committee. (2005) Helping families raise children with special needs at home. *Pediatrics* **115**: 507–511.

Joseph Rowntree Foundation. (1998) Independent Visitors and Disabled Young People. In: *Findings, January 1998 – Ref 138*. York: Joseph Rowntree Foundation. (http://www.jrf.org.uk/knowledge/findings/social care/scr138.asp)

Kennedy M. (1990) The deaf child who was sexually abused – is there a need for a dual specialist? *Child Abuse Rev* **4**: 3–6.

Khan J, Stuart J. (2000) *Second Analysis of Quality Protects Management Action Plans: Services for Disabled Children and their Families*. London: Council for Disabled Children.

Knight A. (1998) *Valued or Forgotten? Independent Visitors and Disabled Young People*. London: National Children's Bureau.

Laan NMA, Loots GMP, Janssen CGCJ, Stalk J. (2001) Foster Care for children with mental retardation and challenging behaviour: a follow-up study. *Brit J Dev Disab* **47**: 3–13.

Local Government Association, Department of Children, Schools and Families, Improvement and Development Agency (forthcoming). *Narrowing the Gap*. London: LGA.

Loughran F, Parker R, Gordon D.(1992). *Children with Disabilities in Communal Establishments: A Further Analysis and Interpretation of the OPCS Investigation*. Bristol: Department of Social Policy and Social Planning, University of Bristol.

Lyon C, Pimor A. (2004) *Physical Interventions and the Law*. Kidderminster: British Institute of Learning Disabilities.

McCann JB, James A, Wilson S, Dunn G. (1996) Prevalence of psychiatric disorders in young people in the care system. *BMJ* **313**: 1529–1530.

McConkey R, Nixon T, Donaghy E, Mulhearn D. (2004) The characteristics of children living away from home and their future service needs. *Br J Soc Work* **34**: 561–576.

McGill P, Tennyson A, Cooper V. (2006) Parents whose children with learning disabilities and challenging behaviour attend 52-week residential schools: their perceptions of services received and expectations of the future. *Br J Soc Work* **36**: 597–616.

Mather M. (2000) Health issues for Black and minority ethnic children. *J Adoption Fostering* **24**: 68–70.

Mather M, Humphrey J, Robson J. (1997) The statutory medical and health needs of looked after children: Time for a radical review? *J Adoption Fostering* **21**: 36–40.

Meltzer H, Corbin T, Gatward R, Goodman R, Ford T. (2003) *The Mental Health of Young People Looked After by Local Authorities in England*. Office of National Statistics. London, The Stationery Office.

Mencap. (2001) *No Ordinary Life*. London: Mencap.

Mencap. (2003) *Breaking Point*. London: Mencap.

Mental Heath Foundation (MHF). (1999) *Bright Futures. Promoting Children and Yong Peoples Mental Health*. London: MHF.

Middleton L. (1992) *Children First: Working with Children and Disability*. Birmingham: Venture Press.

Miller D. (2002) *Disabled Children and Abuse*. NSPCC Information Briefings, February 2002. (http://www.nspcc.org.uk/inform)

Morris J. (1995) *Gone Missing? A Research and Policy Review of Disabled Children Living Away from their Families*. London: Who Cares? Trust.

Morris J. (1998) *Still Missing? Volumes 1 and 2*. London: Who Cares? Trust.

Morris J. (1999) Disabled children, child protection systems and the Children Act 1989. *Child Abuse Rev* **8**: 91–108.

Morris J. (2002) A Lot to Say: A Guide for Social Workers, Personal Advisors and Others Working with Disabled Children and Young People with Communication Impairments. London: Scope.

Morris J, Abbott D, Ward L. (2002) At home or away? An exploration of policy and practice in the placement of disabled children at residential schools. *Children & Society* **16**: 3–16.

National Care Standards Commission. (2004) *How Do We Care? The Availability of Registered Care Homes and Children's Homes and their Performance against National Minimum Standards 2002–03*. London: National Care Standards Commission.

National Working Group on Child Protection and Disability. (2003) *"It Doesn't Happen to Disabled Children": Child Protection and Disabled Children*. London: NSPCC.

Nelson C, Zeanah C, Fox N. (2007) The effects of early intervention on brain-behavioural development. In: Romer D, Walker E, editors. *Adolescent Psycholpathology and the Developing Brain. Integrating Brain and Prevention Science*. Oxford: Oxford University Press.

Office for National Statistics (ONS). (2004) National Statistics Online: *The Health of Children and Young People*. March 2004. (http://www.statistics.gov.uk/children/)

Oliver M. (1990) *The Politics of Disablement*. Basingstoke: The Macmillan Press.

Oswin M. (1991) *They Keep Going Away*. London: King's Fund Publishing. Ch 3, pp 53–86.

Owen M. (1999) *Novices, Old Hands and Professionals: Adoption by Single People*. London: BAAF.

Paul A, Cawson P. (2002) Safeguarding disabled children in residential settings: what we know and what we don't know. *Child Abuse Rev* **11**: 262–281.

Paul A, Cawson P, Paton J. (2004) *Safeguarding Disabled Children in Residential Special Schools*. London: NSPCC.

Payne H, Butler I. (1988) Improving the health care process and determining health outcomes for children looked after by the local authority. *Ambulatory Child Health* **4**: 165–172.

Phillips J. (1997) Meeting the Psychiatric needs of children in foster care. *Psychiatric Bull* **21**: 609–611.

Pithouse A, Hill-Tout J, Lowe K. (2002) Training foster carers in challenging behaviour: a case study in disappointment? *Child Family Social Work* **7**: 1365–2206.

Protection of Children Act 1999. London: The Stationery Office. (http://www.opsi.gov.uk/ACTS/acts1999/ukpga_19990014_en_1)

Quinton D. (2004) Studies of foster care. In: *Supporting Parents: Messages from Research*. London: Jessica Kingsley.

Richardson J and Joughin C. (2000) *Mental Health Needs of Looked After Children*. London: Gaskell.

Richardson M, West MA, Day P, Stuart S. (1989) Children with developmental disabilities in the child welfare system – a national survey. *Child Welfare* **68**: 605–613.

Rick S, Douglas D. (2007) Neurobiological effects of childhood abuse. *J Psychosoc Nurs Men Health Serv* **45**: 47–54.

Robinson C, Weston C, Minkes J. (1995) *Making Progress: Change and Development in Services to Disabled Children under the Children Act 1989*. Bristol: Norah Fry Research Centre, University of Bristol.

Russell, P (1995) The importance of contact for children with disabilities – Issues for policy and practice. In: Argent H, editor. *See You Soon: Contact with Children Looked After by Local Authorities*. London: BAAF.

Rutter, M. (1999) Psychosocial adversity and child psychopathology. *Br J Psychiatry* **174**: 480–493.

Rutter M, and the English and Romanian adoptee (ERA) study team. (1998) Developmental catch-up, and deficit, following adoption after severe global early privation. *J Child Psychol Psychiatry* **39**: 465–476.

Santosh P, Baird G. (1999) Psychopharmacotherapy in children and adults with intellectual disability. *Lancet* **35**: 233–242.

Selwyn J, Sturgess W, Quinton D, Baxter C. (2006) *Costs and Outcomes of Non-infant Adoptions*. London: BAAF.

Sibert JR, Horrocks L, Ranton B. 2002 *Literature Review on Children with Special Health Needs in Wales*. Cardiff: Department of Child Health, University of Wales College of Medicine.

References

Sinclair I, Wilson K. Matches and mismatches: the contribution of carers and children to the success of foster placements. *Br J Soc Work* **33**: 871–884.

Skuse T, Ward H. (1999) *Current Research Findings About the Health of Looked After Children.* Paper for Quality Protects seminar: Improving Health Outcomes for Looked After Children. Dartington Social Research Unit and Loughborough University.

Skuse T, MacDonald I, Ward H. (2001) *Looking After Children: Transforming Data into Management Information. Report of a Longitudinal Study at 30/9/99, Third Interim Report to the Department of Health.* Loughborough: Loughborough University.

Smith R, Policy, Research and Influencing Unit. (2002) *Promoting Children's Emotional Health.* Ilford: Barnados.

Social Exclusion Unit. (2003) *A Better Education for Children in Care.* London: SEU. Social Exclusion Unit. (2004) *Breaking the Cycle.* London: SEU.

Stalker K, Carpenter J, Phillips R et al. (2003) *Care and Treatment? Supporting Children with Complex Needs in Healthcare Settings.* Brighton: Pavilion.

Stanley N, Riordan D, Alaszewski H. (2005) The mental helath of looked after children: matching reesponse to need. *Health Soc Care Community* **13**: 239–248.

Stuart M, Baines C. (2004a) *Safeguards for Vulnerable Children: Three Studies on Abusers, Disabled Children and Children in Prison.* York: Joseph Rowntree Foundation

Stuart M, Baines C. (2004b) *Progress on Safeguards for Children Living Away from Home: A Review of Action since the People Like Us Report.* York: Joseph Rowntree Foundation.

Sullivan P, Knutson J. (1998) The association between child maltreatment and disabilities in a hospital-based epidemiological study. *Child Abuse and Neglect* **22**: 271–288.

Sullivan P, Knutson J. (2000) Maltreatment and disabilities: a population-based epidemiological study. *Child Abuse and Neglect* **24**: 1257–1273.

Support Force for Children's Residential Care. (1995) *Residential Care for Children and Young People: A Positive Choice? Final report to the Secretary of State for Health.* London: DH.

Szymanski LS, Seppala HT. (1995) Specialized family care for children with developmental disabilities: the Finnish experience. *Child Welfare* **74**: 367–381.

Teicher MH, Tomoda A, Anderson, SL. (2006) Neurobiological consequences of early stress and childhood maltreatment: Are results from human and animal studies comparable? *Ann N Y Acad Sci* **821**: 160–175.

Timms JE, Thorburn J. (2003) *Your Shout! A Survey of the Views of 706 Children and Young People in the Public Care.* London: NSPCC.

Triseloitis J, Borland M, and Hill M. (1999). *Delivering Foster Care.* London: BAAF.

Tudor Hart J. (1971) The inverse care law. *Lancet* **1**: 405–412.

United Kingdom Government. (1998) *The Government's Response to the Children's Safeguards Review.* London: The Stationery Office. (http://www.archive.official-documents.co.uk/document/cm41/4105/4105.htm)

United States of America Congress. Adoption and Safe Families Act of 1997. (http://www.acf.hhs.gov/programs/cb/laws_policies/cblaws/public_law/pl105_89/pl105_89.htm)

Utting W. (1997) *People Like Us: The Report of the Review of the Safeguards for Children Living Away from Home.* London: The Stationery Office.

van Ijzendoorn M, Rutgers AH, Bakermans-Kranenburg MJ et al. (2007) Parental sensitivity and attachment in children with autism spectrum disorder: Comparison with children with mental retardation, with language delays and with typical development. *Child Dev* **78**: 597–608.

Waldman HB, Perlman SP. (2004) Female dental practitioners and care of special needs children. *J Dent Chil (Chic)* **71**: 218–221.

Weiler H, Fischer H, Guggenbichler JP, Krautgartner G. (1988) Heilpädagogische Pflegefamilien. Ein Modell zur Rehabilitation behinderter Kinder aus Risikofamilien. *Pädiatrie und Pädologie* **23**: 185–193.

Weinberg LA. (1997) Problems in educating abused and neglected children with disabilities. *Child Abuse Neglect* **21**: 889–905.

Welsh Assembly Government. (2007) Towards a Stable Life and A Brighter Future. London: The Stationery Office. (http://new.wales.gov.uk/docrepos/40382/dhss/510356/1549274?lang=en)

Westcott H. (1991) The abuse of disabled children: a review of the literature. *Child Care Health Dev* **17**: 243–258.

Westcott H. (1993) *The Abuse of Children and Adults with Disabilities.* London: NSPCC.

Westcott H. (1998) Disabled children and child protection. In: Robinson C, Stalker, K editors. *Growing Up with Disability.* London: Jessica Kingsley.

Westcott H, Jones D. (1999) The abuse of disabled children. *J Child Psychol Psychiatry* **40**: 497–506.

Williams J, Jackson S, Maddocks A, Cheung WY, Love A, Hutchings H. (2001) Case control study of the health of those looked after by local authorities. *Arch Dis Child* **85**: 280–285.

Winn Oakley M, Masson J. (2000) *Official Friends and Friendly Officials: Support, advice and advocacy for children and young people in public care.* London: NSPCC.

Wolpert M, Fuggle P, Cottrell D et al. (2002) *Drawing on the Evidence: Advice for Mental Health Professionals working with Children and Adolescents.* London: The British Psychological Society.

Wright V. (2004) Case study: A consultant nurse for looked after children. *Prof Nurse* **20**: 26.

Index

Index